The Jewish Pregnancy Book

A Resource for the Soul, Body & Mind during Pregnancy, Birth & the First Three Months

Sandy Falk, M.D., and Rabbi Daniel Judson

with Steven A. Rapp

JEWISH LIGHTS Publishing

Woodstock, Vermont

The Jewish Pregnancy Book:
A Resource for the Soul, Body & Mind during Pregnancy, Birth & the First Three Months

2004 First Printing

Library of Congress Cataloging-in-Publication Data
Falk, Sandy, 1968–
The Jewish pregnancy book : a resource for the soul, body & mind during pregnancy, birth & the first three months / Sandy Falk and Rabbi Daniel Judson with Steven A. Rapp.

      p. cm.
Includes bibliographical references.
ISBN 1-58023-178-0 (pbk.)
1. Pregnancy—Popular works. 2. Pregnancy—Religious aspects—Judaism. 3. Childbirth—Popular works. 4. Childbirth—Religious aspects—Judiasm. 5. Pregnant women—Prayer-books and devotions—English. 6. Jewish women—Prayer-books and devotions—English. 7. Judaism—Prayer-books and devotions—English. I. Judson, Daniel. II. Rapp, Steven A., 1964– III. Title.
RG525.F34 2003
618.2—dc22
2003018799

10 9 8 7 6 5 4 3 2 1

Manufactured in the United States of America

Published by Jewish Lights Publishing
A Division of LongHill Partners, Inc.
Sunset Farm Offices, Route 4, P.O. Box 237
Woodstock, VT 05091
Tel: (802) 457-4000   Fax: (802) 457-4004
www.jewishlights.com

To my mother, Bruria Bodek Falik, with love and gratitude. May every child be blessed with a parent for whom her heart cries out, and is always answered.

—S.F.

To my mother, Betty Judson, who loved being pregnant so much that she had many children, each of whom is blessed to have her worry, her respect, and her love.

—D.J.

To my mother, Anita W. Rapp, of blessed memory, who carried me for nine months and beyond.

—S.R.

Contents

<u>6</u>

From This Narrow Place I Call to You:
Pregnancy Loss 103

A Synagogue Ritual for Miscarriage • One Hundred and Eighty Degrees: A Miscarriage

<u>7</u>

Aleph-Bet Yoga for Pregnancy 111

Yoga for Overall Well-Being during Pregnancy • What Is Yoga? • Why Practice Yoga during Pregnancy • Yoga for Each Stage of Your Pregnancy • Yoga for the Jewish Soul • Getting Ready to Practice • How to Practice the Aleph-Bet Yoga Series • Cautionary Notes for Practicing Yoga during Pregnancy • The Aleph-Bet Yoga Poses • What Is the Correct Order for Practicing Aleph-Bet Yoga during Each Trimester? • Guidelines for a Shorter Session

---

Cautionary Note for Practicing Yoga during Pregnancy

During the first trimester and first two months following delivery, you should avoid practicing certain Aleph-Bet Yoga poses; others should be avoided during second and third trimesters. For specific information see pages 127–130. Also, before starting or continuing a yoga practice while pregnant, you should consult with your physician.

Acknowledgments

We would like to thank Stuart M. Matlins, publisher of Jewish Lights, for believing that there is no life-cycle event that Judaism cannot enhance and enrich. We would also like to thank Emily Wichland, managing editor at Jewish Lights, and our editor, Donna Zerner. Donna's meticulous reading of the manuscript with both her mind and her soul was invaluable.

We were blessed to work with Steven Rapp as our coauthor. Steve's writing reflects his personality—kind, open, gentle, and wise. Dan has been honored to have Steve as a congregant and as a teacher. He is a gifted poet, a talented yoga teacher (even for the inflexible among us), a spiritually vibrant soul, and—perhaps most important—a true mensch.

We would also like to thank those authors who wrote a poem or a story for this project: Rabbi Amy Bardack, Joanna Selznick Dulkin, Amy Friedman, Franci Levine Grater, Martha Hausman, Rabbi Dianne Cohler-Esses, Aurora Mendelsohn, Rabbi Michelle Robinson, Rabbi Sandy Eisenberg Sasso, Rabbi Susan Silverman, Sandy Slavet, Rabbi Shira Stern, and Rabbi Shohama Wiener.

We are grateful to Rabbi Amy Bardack and Naomi Rush for their insightful comments on the manuscript.

Rabbis Marjorie Slome, Barbara Penzner, and Rifat Sonsino were helpful in providing resources for sections of the book.

Finally, we would like to thank Naftali Lev Falk-Judson, the inspiration for this book and the daily joy of our lives.

Sandy Falk
Dan Judson

I would like to thank Sandy Falk and Dan Judson for inviting me to collaborate on this special project. I especially want to thank Ulrike Rapp and Abby Jacob (and Kennedy) for modeling so beautifully for the yoga photos. Similarly, a big thanks to photographer Steven Lewis for his artistic eye and skillful work. Special thanks to the JFK Fitness Center and its members for providing the space to take the photographs. And finally, profound thanks to my mother and all the women in my family, who carried my ancestors and, in doing so, carried me to this moment.

Steven Rapp

Introduction

When people ask each of us what our spouse does, and we answer that we are an obstetrician and a rabbi, we often get comments such as, "Oh, a doctor and a rabbi, a marriage of opposites. One of you deals with the body, while the other deals with the soul." When it comes to pregnancy, however, an obstetrician and a rabbi are not opposites. Pregnancy encompasses both body and soul. When Sandy was pregnant and reached the final weeks of her pregnancy, we were very conscious of the fact that she could go into labor at any time. There was an unpredictability that felt like she was sitting in the palm of God's hand. Pregnancy is a miraculous and challenging process of creation. It is a partnership between a woman, her partner, her doctor or midwife, and God.

If you are picking up this book, you probably already regard pregnancy and birth as a spiritual experience. In the past few years, more and more women are coming to see their pregnancy not simply as a physical experience to be endured, but as a spiritually meaningful period in their life. This book provides a wealth of Jewish resources to enrich and enhance your experience of pregnancy.

There is only one small problem. The talmudic Rabbis, who formulated the basis of traditional Jewish prayer, ritual, and law, were men. And because they were men, they never experienced pregnancy. The Rabbis never felt the disquiet of morning sickness, never endured the discomfort of trying to sleep with a huge belly, and never had their bodies enveloped by labor pains. As Blu Greenberg, the orthodox Jewish feminist, noted, the Rabbis' maleness may account for the dearth of prayers, rituals, and blessings that Judaism has for pregnancy and delivery. The Rabbis were very detail-oriented: They created blessings for many events, such as a blessing for before and after eating, a blessing for seeing someone who looked unusual, a blessing for smelling a fragrant tree, a blessing for hearing bad news, even a blessing for buying new clothes. And so it is quite striking that the Rabbis "skipped" this entire passage of life. If the Rabbis were women, Blu Greenberg speculates, there would probably be some fantastic birthing rituals.[1]

In recent years, Jewish women have been trying to make up for this silence by creating their own pregnancy prayers and rituals. Women have also searched the cobwebs of Jewish tradition to find prayers that our foremothers passed from one generation to the next. In this book, we continue the process of creating Jewish prayers and rituals and include some traditional ones as well. We also provide other resources beyond rituals and prayers. This book is for the whole being: the mind, body, and soul of a pregnant Jewish woman.

For your mind, we have basic medical information on topics such as fetal development, morning sickness, genetic testing, and the stages of labor. Interwoven with this medical information are traditional and contemporary Jewish sources on these subjects. This book also offers the Jewish perspective on a number of ethical issues that may arise during your pregnancy, such as selective reduction and prenatal testing.

For your body, we have prenatal Aleph-Bet Yoga, a unique blend of yoga and the Hebrew letters created by Steven Rapp, author of *Aleph-Bet Yoga: Embodying the Hebrew Letters for Physical and Spiritual Well-Being* (Jewish Lights). Aleph-Bet Yoga is a method of moving your body through hatha yoga poses that approximate letters of the Hebrew *aleph-bet*. A prenatal yoga practice is an ideal way for a woman to prepare physically for the one of the most challenging athletic events of her life. A regimen of yoga may mean less physical discomfort, less stress, and more energy for an easier pregnancy and an easier labor. Aleph-Bet prenatal yoga is designed to help your body gently carry your pregnancy and ready itself for delivery. The poses are suitable for beginners as well as intermediate yoga practitioners.

Aleph-Bet Yoga provides more than just physical benefits, though. By forming the Hebrew letters, you focus on the deeper meaning of those letters, providing a spiritual connection to your physical workout. The Hebrew letters are considered by Jewish mystical tradition to be a gateway to God's presence; they are holy vessels carrying the light of God. By embodying the Hebrew letters, you will be tapping into this light and letting it flow through you and your fetus.

For your soul, we provide prayers, rituals, and *kavvanot* (intentions) for each stage of pregnancy. Some of the prayers are centuries old but have only recently come to light, such as the prayer for every day of pregnancy from an eighteenth-century Italian *siddur* (prayer book) for a married woman. Some of the prayers are psalms that have traditionally been associated with labor. And some of the prayers have been written recently, such as the prayer for morning sickness—yes, we have a prayer for morning sickness, because Judaism understands that there is no aspect of life that is outside God's blessings.

Even if you do not pray regularly, we invite you to experiment with the prayers found in this book. We suggest taking a few moments of quiet before saying any of the prayers, be conscious of saying them slowly, focusing on the words and allowing your mind to fill with the images the prayers present.

We also include some personal reflections and stories about pregnancy from women who have drawn on Judaism's spiritual resources to help them through difficult periods. Rabbi Amy Bardack describes her experience of saying *Birkat Hagomel* (the blessing for safe deliverance from danger) after experiencing preeclampsia, a potentially fatal disease related to pregnancy. Franci Levine Grater describes her experience of having premature twins in the Neonatal Intensive Care Unit (NICU) and the blessings she recited for their safety. We hope these personal stories will help you prepare for the roller coaster of pregnancy.

Finally, this book provides a wealth of traditional Jewish sources on the nature of pregnancy. We include some biblical material, some material culled from Jewish mystical tradition, and a large amount of material from rabbinic sources. The Rabbis had a different concept of the physical processes of pregnancy and a different understanding of the role of women in society than our contemporary society holds, yet their understanding of God has been the focal point of Judaism for the past two millennia. So while we acknowledge that their words may not have as much medical or sociological validity for us today, we believe that their writings about pregnancy still hold profound spiritual insight.

We should note that this book is not meant as the sole medical resource you use for your pregnancy. It is a companion book. The medical information we provide does not cover every topic related to pregnancy, but if you are like many pregnant women, having two, three, or even six books about pregnancy is not unusual. This book is a uniquely Jewish enhancement to your collection.

We hope that you will use this book as a spiritual resource as you make your way from pregnancy to birth and beyond, and we hope that your entire being—body, mind, and soul—will be nourished by the pages that follow. We offer this blessing as a beginning for your journey:

May your experience of pregnancy and birth be healthy, joyful, and filled with awe.

1

The First Trimester

You're Pregnant! *B'sha-ah Tovah!*

The moment you find out you are pregnant is life-changing. You may have been trying to conceive for months or years, or perhaps this is a less-than-expected event. This incredible news may make you jump for joy; it may set your head spinning with the panic of wondering how in the world you are going to be able to raise a child. I know that we took a picture of the test kit to prove to ourselves that it was real. Many women see their doctor after a positive home pregnancy test and ask for a "real test" to check. Guess what, you really *are* pregnant! The doctor's test is the same as the home test. Still, some news merits repeating, and I am sure that your doctor will be happy to do a test for you.

When and how you decide to share the news with others is a personal choice. Many people wait for a few months to tell friends and family, both to become comfortable privately with the idea of parenthood and to feel confident that the pregnancy will continue. Of course, some people are on the phone with their mother seconds after the two little stripes appear on the pregnancy test screen.

When you do share your news with others, you may find that your Jewish friends and relatives say, "*B'sha-ah tovah,*" which literally means, "in a good hour." You may have been expecting the more familiar Jewish congratulatory expression, *mazel tov*. But there is a reason why the phrase *b'sha-ah tovah* is used. Our Jewish culture is a cautious one, and pregnancy is considered a liminal state, a state of potentiality. Hopefully you will have a wonderful pregnancy and give birth to a healthy baby. But Judaism understands that where there is potential for joy, there is also potential for loss. So Jewish superstition tells us not to say *mazel tov*, congratulations, until the process is done and you are holding a healthy baby in your arms. Instead, we say *b'sha-ah tovah*, a phrase that has an astrological connotation to it, meaning, "May the baby be born safely in a good hour when the planets are aligned in a fortuitous way."

A Prayer upon Learning of a Pregnancy

When the biblical Sarah learns that she is pregnant, she laughs in amazement to herself. The Torah tells us that she had already stopped menstruating, and she does not believe that she is capable of becoming pregnant. In response to her laughter, God says, "Is anything too wondrous for the Lord?"(Genesis 18:13). Indeed, even without the special circumstances of Sarah, you may find yourself laughing at how unfathomable it is to give life to another human being. The Talmud understands that every pregnancy is a wondrous act of God. It teaches that there are three partners in the creation of a human being: the mother, the father, and God (*Niddah* 31a).

In gratitude to God, as well as in the hope that the pregnancy will be healthy, Rabbi Sandy Eisenberg Sasso offers the following prayer to be recited upon learning of a pregnancy:

(Before saying this prayer, sit for a moment with your eyes closed, and open your heart to welcoming the new soul you have created.)

Prayer upon Discovering the News

[Partners together:]

We stand breathless before the Power of Creation that works through us to bring forth new life. We tremble with fear and joy.

[*Pregnant woman:*]

Deep inside me a seed is growing. I am afraid, and I am filled with ecstasy.

[*Partners together:*]

May this promise of life come to be—our child. We trust in the source of life, this power which grips us within and yet transcends us. Protect this fragile new beginning. May we find love and strength to nurture this gift of fertility and life. Sheltered under wings of love, may we grow to be partners with the source of life in the miracle of creation.

בָּרוּךְ אַתָּה יְיָ אֱלֹהֵינוּ מֶלֶךְ הָעוֹלָם,
שֶׁהֶחֱיָנוּ וְקִיְּמָנוּ וְהִגִּיעָנוּ לַזְּמַן הַזֶּה.

Barukh ata Adonai, eloheinu melekh ha'olam,
shehecheyanu, v'kiyimanu, v'higiyanu, lazman hazeh.

Blessed by the presence whose sanctity fills our lives, we give thanks for life, health, and this sacred moment.

Conception

A friend of ours, Shana, claims that she knew the moment her daughter was conceived. "It just felt special; my husband and I just connected so deeply when we were making love that I knew that was the night and thought I could even feel the conception physically." Shana feels that her daughter was marked for good things because the moment of her conception was such a wonderful experience.

There are many Jewish stories that reflect similar thinking, that the thoughts and feelings of the parents at the time of conception directly affect the fetus. The Talmud tells the story of a man who is very careful to think only of his wife and no other woman when they are trying to conceive so that the fetus can receive blessings (*Nedarim* 20b). The Talmud also states that negative thoughts will have a detrimental effect on the fetus. It says that if conception occurs when someone is intoxicated or if there is hatred between the couple, the child will be thought of as a rebel against God (*Nedarim* 20b). Bachya ben Asher, a fourteenth-century commentator on the Torah, says that when a husband and wife have intercourse to conceive, they must purge their minds of impure thoughts of other people. The degree of their moral and spiritual purity will affect the soul of their fetus (R. Bachya on Genesis 30:39).

The Talmud takes this idea even further, saying that what the parents are thinking during sex can affect not only the character of the fetus but the physical makeup as well. There is a story in the Talmud of the king of Arabia (who was dark-skinned) having a fair-skinned child, and so he accuses his wife (who is also dark-skinned) of having had an affair. The king consults with Rabbi Akiva, who suggests that his wife might have been looking at a white statue in the room at the time of conception, which thus caused the white baby (*Genesis Rabbah* 73:10).

The Rabbis also understood that at the moment of conception, the sex of the fetus was determined. This was based on who "gave forth seed" (had an orgasm) first. If the man gives forth seed first, then the baby will be a girl; if the woman puts forth seed first, then the baby will be a boy. The Rabbis further say that because the sex is determined at conception, there is no point in praying for a specific gender after conception has happened (*Berakhot* 60a). The Rabbis are against praying to God for things that we know are already determined.

Although the Rabbis did not know the biological facts, they were correct in their belief that sex was determined at the moment of conception. From what we now know about chromosomes, it is remarkable, really, how much is determined at the instant of conception. In some ways, the moment of conception is the most important moment of your life; it is too bad we aren't aware of it. Everything from eye color to gender to potential genetic problems is determined in that one split second. And yet at the same time that so much has already been decided, none of it is known to us. So while the Rabbis say one should not pray for the gender of the fetus after the fact, they say that every day a prayer should be recited so that the fetus remains healthy and develops normally.

Morning Sickness

Pregnancy is a total body experience. Within several weeks of finding out that you are pregnant, you may come to this realization with the onset of "morning sickness." You may soon start to feel that pregnancy-related nausea and vomiting should be more accurately renamed "all-day sickness."

The cause of this condition, which is called "hyperemesis gravidarum" in its most severe form, is not clearly understood. You are not alone; 70 percent of women experience this to some degree.[2] One important element may be the effect of the hormone progesterone, which relaxes the muscles of the internal organs. Progesterone is at a high level in a pregnant woman and this causes relaxation of the stomach, which may contribute to nausea and to an increased tendency toward vomiting. This also accounts for the common experience of heartburn and constipation in pregnancy. Estrogens may also play a role. Another factor may be a response to hCG, since the typical timing of these symptoms correlates with the rise and fall of hCG in early pregnancy. On the bright side, pregnant women affected by "morning sickness" seem to have lower rates of miscarriage than those who experience no or minimal morning sickness.[3]

The problem may date back to Eve. The Torah says famously that Eve's punishment for eating the apple is to suffer pain during childbirth, but a midrash goes even further. It contends that God's plan for women was that they become pregnant and give birth in one day without any pain, but because Eve ate the apple, women now have to suffer from morning sickness and other pregnancy woes (*Pirkei de Rabbi Eliezer* 14). A period of severe nausea and vomiting can be a very trying time in your pregnancy. If you are experiencing these symptoms, do not feel guilty if you find yourself feeling less than joyful about the pregnancy itself. In the bad old days of medical history, some thought that these symptoms reflected a woman's ambivalence or shame about her pregnancy. We know today that this is not true. This time in your pregnancy can also be difficult for your partner, who may not be sure how to make you feel better. Also, this is the first sign that the pregnancy is physically happening for only one of you.

One concern many women have is that because of their morning sickness they do not eat healthfully. Some women who suffer from nausea find relief only by constantly eating crackers and other carbohydrates; this may lead to weight gain. Other women are not able to keep food down and lose weight. Do not be overly concerned; a fetus can tolerate maternal weight loss or gain in the first trimester.

There are many approaches to treating morning sickness. Dietary modifications, including eating small, frequent, high-carbohydrate meals, help many women. Vitamin B_6 (pyridoxine) supplementation has been found to be effective.[4] Another approach is to apply acupressure to the antinausea pressure points located three finger-widths above the wrist crease.[5] This may be done manually or by wearing wristbands, such as Sea-Band or Relief Band. Ask your doctor or midwife about antinausea medications and other options. Most treatments help lessen the nausea but do not eliminate it completely. Morning sickness usually ends at about fourteen to sixteen weeks.

Ultimately, though, morning sickness is generally a positive signal that the fetus is alive. Within the nausea lies the blessing of this knowledge. Seeing morning sickness as a positive sign may be difficult to keep in mind as you go through your umpteenth box of crackers. There is no traditional blessing for morning sickness. We suggest a prayer modeled after the *asher yatsar* (that created openings) blessing, a daily prayer that acknowledges bodily functions.

In its traditional form, it is recited after first using the bathroom each morning.

When we say the *asher yatsar*, we thank God for keeping all the openings of the body in working order. Judaism understands that all parts of this world are connected to God, and even something like using the bathroom in the morning is a miraculous aspect of God's world that should be blessed. Morning sickness is, of course, different from relieving oneself, but it struck us that the sheer earthiness of the blessing made it useful for this phase of pregnancy. We have adapted the prayer to focus more specifically on pregnancy. The prayer could be said each morning for the duration of your morning sickness:

Prayer for Morning Sickness

Blessed are You, Adonai, our God, ruler of the universe, who created women with wisdom and created within women a womb. It is obvious and known before your throne of glory that if my body was not working properly it would be impossible for this pregnancy to survive. Blessed are You, Adonai, who heals all flesh and acts wondrously.

Exercise & Diet

Many women ask about exercise during pregnancy. The first trimester of pregnancy is not the time to start training for a marathon, but some exercise will help maintain your sense of well-being and may help prepare you for the physical demands of delivery. The rule of thumb is don't start a new high-impact exercise regimen while you are pregnant. If you are already a runner, you may continue to run until it becomes too uncomfortable, usually in the second trimester (consult your physician for advice about your particular situation). If you did not do vigorous exercise before you became pregnant, you probably will want to stick to low-impact exercise. Walking and swimming are often good choices. Many gyms have exercise classes for pregnant women. Another favorite for pregnancy is yoga. The last chapter of this book is devoted to Aleph-Bet prenatal yoga by Steven Rapp; these routines offer both physical and spiritual enrichment for your pregnancy.

In terms of diet, the general recommendation for a pregnant woman is to gain between twenty-five and thirty-five pounds. There are special circumstances where this number changes, such as carrying multiple fetuses, but in general you should be cognizant of this general range. There is some risk associated with not gaining at least twenty pounds over the course of the pregnancy because low weight gain can negatively affect the fetus's growth. Going over the weight limit poses less of a problem. Women have gained seventy pounds or more and had a perfectly healthy baby. Weight gain over this range may lead to a larger fetus, though this is not always the case.

Before modern nutrition, the Rabbis of the Talmud had their own idea of what a pregnant woman should eat. They said that meat and wine should be eaten for a robust baby and too much liquor would cause an ungainly child. Eggs should be eaten for eyesight, fish for gracefulness, parsley for beauty, coriander for stoutness, and *etrog* for fragrance. The Rabbis warn against eating mustard, believed to cause gluttonous children, and fish brine and cress, thought to harm the eyes. The Rabbis also warn against eating clay, which will cause ugliness (*Ketubot* 60b–71a). A midrash says that the dietary needs of a pregnant woman needed to be taken into account even during the hurried Exodus from Egypt. When God commanded Moses to take the Israelites out of Egypt, one of Moses' concerns was food, so he asked God: "Have You [God] also prepared *rekikin* (soft foods) for the pregnant women, *anonas* [provisions] for the nursing mothers...?" (*Exodus Rabbah* 3:4).

Cravings

Pregnant women often have intense cravings for certain foods. These cravings actually have a famous place in Jewish law. The Rabbis of the Talmud give a special dispensation from fasting for women who are suffering from these cravings on Yom Kippur. The Rabbis say, "If a pregnant woman smells a dish and becomes faint because of a desire for it on the Day of Atonement [Yom Kippur], she must be given it to eat until she feels restored" (*Yoma* 8:5).

This may seem fairly straightforward; if a pregnant woman is ravenous, feed her even on the most important fast day of the year. But the rabbinic mind is never satisfied with a simple answer. The Rabbis further ask about the situation in which a pregnant woman craves a food that is *treyf* (nonkosher). Can you eat pork on Yom Kippur if you crave it? The Rabbis say that one should first remind the woman that it is Yom Kippur, then try to give the women a piece of food dipped in the juice of the prohibited meat. If this does not alleviate the craving, then indeed the woman should be given the nonkosher food until her craving is satiated (*Yoma* 82b).

The reason the Rabbis give for allowing a pregnant woman to eat pork on Yom Kippur is that observing the commandments should not impair a person's health. The Rabbis presumed it was medically unsafe for the woman if she did not satisfy her cravings. Although modern medicine does not believe that letting cravings go unsatisfied will cause any real harm, it may at times certainly feel to you (and your partner) that satisfying a craving is critical to your survival.

Fetal Development in the First Trimester

The Rabbis were astonished by the physiology of pregnancy. "Come and see the miraculous ways of God. When a human being turns a keg of water over so that its opening is facing downward, all the water contained in it would spill it. But God puts the fetus in the womb with the opening facing downward and it does not spill out" (*Niddah* 31a).

The Rabbis, living in the first millennium, had a different view of fetal development than we do now. Although we would not look to them for accurate medical knowledge, their view of fetal development has its own wisdom concerning God's role in the womb.

A midrash describes the rabbinic understanding of conception. It says that the uterus is always full of red blood, some of which comes out as menstrual blood during a woman's period. When it is God's will, a drop of white substance (sperm) falls in and immediately a fetus begins to form. The fetus may be compared to milk in a basin. If one puts rennet into it, it congeals and becomes solid; if not, it continues as liquid (*Leviticus Rabbah* 13:9). The Talmud says that from the white of the father are derived the fetus's bones and sinews, the nails, the marrow in the bone, and the white of the eye. From the red of the mother are derived the skin, the flesh, the blood, the hair, and the black of the eye. God gives the soul, the beauty of features, sight of the eyes, hearing of the ears, speech of the mouth, the ability to move the hands and walk with the feet, and understanding and discernment. When the time arrives for a person to depart from this world, God takes God's portion back and leaves the portions contributed by the parents (*Niddah* 31a).

After conception, the Rabbis offer a few different opinions as to how the fetus develops. Some Rabbis believe that God forms the fetus completely right after conception. In another discussion however, Rabbi Ishmael claims that the male fetus is fully developed after forty-one days in the womb, while the female fetus is fully developed after eighty-one days. Most of the Rabbis believe that a fetus of either sex is fully formed after forty-one days (*Niddah* 30b).

Interestingly, like the rabbinic view of embryonic development, the modern scientific understanding of this process also includes the formation of the fetus from three preexistent sources. After the egg and sperm meet, the developing conceptus, known for the first two weeks as a zygote, begins dividing itself into ever-growing numbers of cells. These cells ultimately fan out into layers, forming the initial basis of the placenta and the fetus. Weeks three through eight are the embryonic stage, during which all the major organ systems develop. The blueprint for this process includes the development of three distinct cell layers, much like the three sources of the body envisioned by our forbears. These three layers are the endoderm, which will become the digestive and respiratory systems; the mesoderm, source of the muscles, bones, deeper layers of the skin, heart, kidneys, and gonads; and the ectoderm, which will develop into the nervous system and the surface of the skin.

Ensoulment

In Jewish tradition, a prayer recited every morning says, "God, the soul that You have given me is a pure one." Judaism understands that we each have a soul, a life force given to us by God. A midrash describes how God actually created all the souls of all human beings in the six days of creation; when a child is born, a soul is put into his or her body. "Know that all the souls, those that existed since Adam and those that will still come into being until the end of the whole world, were created in the six days of Creation, and were all in the Garden of Eden, and all were present at the giving of the Torah" (Tanchuma, *Pekude* 3).

The *Zohar*, Judaism's classic mystical text, holds a slightly different understanding. The *Zohar* says that God created all the souls that are to be born into the world, but each of these souls has a male and female aspect to it. When the soul descends into the world, the male and female aspects split apart and go into different bodies. God knows which male soul was initially matched with each female soul, and God brings them together later in marriage (*Zohar* I, 85b). From this idea we get the Jewish concept of *bashert*, one's destined partner. The *Zohar* says that we have been destined for a partner, the other half of our soul, not only from the day we were born, but also from the very beginning of time, when all the souls were created. (How's that for pressure?)

The question of when the soul enters the body is actually not given great weight in rabbinic Judaism. There is in fact only one explicit discussion of this question in all of rabbinic literature. A

Greek ruler and philosopher named Antoninus asked a rabbi, "At which stage is the soul instilled in man?"[6] Said the rabbi to him, "As soon as he leaves his mother's womb [is born]." He (Antoninus) replied, "If you leave meat unsalted for three days will it not become putrid [as soon as the fetus is conceived, must not the soul be added to it like salt to meat or it will not remain viable]?" (*Genesis Rabbah* 34:10). The argument began with the rabbi believing that the soul becomes part of the body only at birth, but the rabbi changed his mind and accepted the answer that the soul enters the body at conception. It should be noted, however, that the Greek philosopher originated this idea. That is to say that Judaism accepts the idea, not as the result of the usual process of talmudic debate, but almost as an afterthought from a foreign thinker. It has been posited that the Rabbis are not so concerned with the exact moment of ensoulment because Judaism does not believe in the strict separation between the soul and the body that marks much of Christian thought.[7]

The question of when the soul enters the body is crucial in today's religious debate over abortion, however. If the soul enters at conception, then the embryo is a human being, and this of course would have serious implications for abortion rights. The particular issue of ensoulment does not seem to be an important factor in the Jewish debate over the permissibility of abortion (see next chapter for further discussion). As we will see in the next section, the Rabbis believe there is a spiritual life growing in the womb, but they also suggest that the fetus having a soul does not make him/her alive in the same way we are. One well-known scholar in this area suggests that the best way to summarize the rabbinic viewpoint on when ensoulment occurs is that it is a secret belonging to God.[8]

The Spiritual Development of the Fetus

We have friends who, when pregnant, read to their fetus every night. We know other parents who played music for their fetus; they even bought those little pregnancy headphones that go over the pregnant mother's belly. We generally just talked to our fetus. We picked a name for it, making sure it was a very different name than the one it would get outside the womb (we picked an incredibly obscure and difficult to pronounce biblical name for reasons we still do not fathom). We would tell it about our lives and the people who would, with God's help, be a part of its life when it stopped being an "it" and became a he or a she. It happened that Sandy was pregnant during the last year of her obstetrical training, so there were often times when she was under great stress and tremendously sleep deprived, and she would talk to the fetus, telling it just to hang in there. Reading, singing, playing music, and speaking to the growing fetus are all manifestations of the belief that the fetus has an emotional and spiritual life going on inside the womb.

A number of Jewish stories depict the spiritual life of the fetus inside the womb. The most famous of these stories says that the fetus sits in the mother's womb with a light source over its head. The fetus possesses complete wisdom. All is illuminated, and the fetus can see from one end of the world to the other. The fetus learns the entire Torah and discovers what will happen to him/her during the course of his/her life. The fetus is also shown the entire course of human history from the time of creation to the future messianic time when all people will live in peace.

When the time comes for the fetus to enter the world, it protests, not wanting to leave the womb. The fetus is then forced out into the world but comes into it screaming in protest (the baby's first cries). As soon as the baby is born, an angel slaps it above the mouth, creating the indentation between the nose and the mouth, and the baby forgets all the wisdom it learned in the womb.[9] This is somewhat reminiscent of the image of the doctor slapping a newborn baby. This was done to stimulate the baby and help clear out the lungs for a newborn's first breath. By the way, don't worry, this practice is not actually done anymore.

Sex during Pregnancy

The Rabbis of the Talmud have an interesting discussion about sex during pregnancy. We should first note that, although the Rabbis understand the primary function of sex as procreation, they also acknowledge sexual activity purely for pleasure. The Rabbis' discussion centers around their understanding of anatomy. They believe that the womb is divided into lower, middle, and upper compartments. Their understanding is that the fetus is in the lowest compartment for the first trimester and in the middle compartment for the second semester. In the final trimester, the fetus is in the upper chamber, where it turns over, head down, to come out. They believed the act of turning downward to be the source of labor pains.

The Rabbis warn against sex during the first trimester but believe it to be beneficial in the third trimester. They write that, because the fetus is in the lowest chamber during the first trimester, the penetration of the male during sexual intercourse could harm the fetus and the mother. They are split about sex during the second trimester, believing it to be dangerous for the mother but beneficial for the fetus. They believe it is beneficial for the fetus because semen gives the fetus vitality. During the last trimester, when the fetus is in the highest chamber, they believe sex is beneficial to both mother and fetus (*Niddah* 31a).

Modern obstetrical advice sounds the same note of caution as the Rabbis regarding sex in the first trimester, though for different reasons. Male semen contains both prostaglandins and oxytocin, hormones that stimulate uterine contractions. If you have a history of pregnancy loss or preterm labor, or are experiencing cramping, bleeding, or fluid leakage from your vagina, you should not have sexual intercourse until you speak with your doctor or midwife. On the other hand, there are no precautions against sex during a healthy pregnancy.

Your desires or positioning may change according to your needs as the pregnancy progresses. As your due date approaches, you may hope for the onset of labor. Having sex in order to induce contractions is one bit of advice that has been passed from woman to woman across the ages. So, if you are beyond thirty-seven weeks, you may just decide to try to use those hormones to your advantage.

Protection against Miscarriage

Miscarriages are common, more common than most women realize. Roughly 30 percent of all pregnancies end in pregnancy loss, with the vast majority occurring in the first trimester.[10] Toward the end of this book, there is a section specifically for those who have suffered pregnancy loss, but we want to include here some Jewish traditions for protecting against miscarriage.

Historically, Jews have offered many explanations for miscarriage. Stories in the Talmud suggest some rather odd causes, such as a very strong wind (*Gittin* 31b) or stepping on fingernails that have been cast into the middle of the street (*Niddah* 17b). The Talmud also suggests that miscarriage is a punishment from God for committing the sin of inciting hatred among people (*Shabbat* 32b). Medieval Jews believed that a woman could miscarry because of excessive leanness or obesity, or as a result of exertion or taking a steambath.[11]

In trying to protect themselves from miscarriage, Jewish women historically turned to charms, amulets, and prayers to gain God's protection. The Talmud records that women wore a stone called an *even tekuma*, a "preserving stone" (*Shabbat* 66b). Later writers suggest that the birthing stone described in the Talmud was an eagle stone, a stone that had a hollow space in it with a loose pebble. Because the stone had another stone within it, it was considered a "pregnant" stone, and thus protective against miscarriage.[12] In addition to the preserving stone, we have historical records of pregnant women carrying with them different verses from Psalms written on parchment, including Psalm 116:6, "The Lord protects the simple; I was brought low, and God saved me," and Psalm 128:3, "Your wife shall be like a fruitful vine…."[13]

Another folk custom, still observed by some women today, is to carry a piece of red thread that has been wrapped around Rachel's (the matriarch) tomb, which is located near Bethlehem. Rachel is connected with pregnancy and pregnancy loss because she pleaded with Jacob to have children and then died during childbirth while delivering Benjamin. A famous midrash about Rachel says that her tears have the power to cause God to act with grace toward Israel. Her connection with pregnancy and divine intervention thus make her a natural focus for prayers to prevent miscarriage. Because most women reading this book will not make it to the tomb of Rachel, we have heard of "regular" red threads being carried by pregnant women, with the symbolic intention that they are threads from Rachel's tomb.

Carrying around psalms or red threads may seem antiquated to some, even heretical to those who see these things as amulets. Nevertheless, at the risk of being called idolaters, we suggest that you consider carrying in your pocket or in a necklace a prayer, a red thread, or even a stone that has personal meaning. While we obviously cannot say whether this will be effective in preserving your fetus, you may benefit from feeling that you are taking an active role in seeking your fetus's safety.

Another way Jewish women sought to protect their fetuses was through daily prayer. In 1786, Yehudit Kutshcer Coen of Italy received from her husband a gift of a prayer book to be used, "especially during her pregnancy, labor and birth, and purification from her (monthly) impurity." In her book *Out of the Depths I Call to You: A Book of Prayers for the Married Jewish Woman*, Rabbi Nina Beth Cardin translates this eighteenth-century Italian prayer book. The following prayer is adapted from this collection. It is meant to be said every day of pregnancy during morning prayers at the conclusion of the *Amidah* (the central prayer of the morning service):

An Eighteenth-Century Prayer
for Every Day of Pregnancy

Lord of the Universe, Ruler of the Hosts, all creatures look hopefully to You. In their time of trouble they look to You for salvation. And even though I am not worthy to come before You with my prayer, I harden my resolve and approach to humbly place my request before You. Just as you remembered Sarah, heeded Rebekah, saw Leah's sorrow, and did not forget Rachel, just as You listened to the voice of all the righteous women when they turned to You, so may You hear the sound of my plea and send the redeeming angel to protect me and to help me throughout my pregnancy.

In accordance with Your graciousness, save me from all harm, sickness, hurt, disability, and pain. Be gracious to me so that the child I carry not be malformed, and grant me an unconditional gift from Your finest treasure trove. Listen to the prayer that springs from the deepest recesses of my heart, and let the child I bear within me be righteous, good, and proper. Strengthen me and gird me so I shall not miscarry.

Be gracious unto me and listen to my prayer, for You listen to the prayers of all who call upon You. Blessed be the One who listens to prayers.[14]

2

The Second Trimester

Dan's mother is a worrier. Like some people breathe, she worries. So for her, as for many expectant parents and grandparents, the first trimester is a time of tension. When we first told Dan's mother about the pregnancy, she told us to call back when we reached the second trimester and she could stop worrying. Having reached the second trimester, your fears of miscarriage should decrease as well. Because 80 percent of miscarriages occur in the first twelve weeks,[1] making it to the second trimester means you have crossed one of pregnancy's biggest hurdles.

The second trimester is often when a pregnant woman feels her best and takes on that pregnancy glow. You will soon feel your baby move for the first time. You will begin to show, and everyone will see that you are pregnant even if you have not said so. This often leads to odd behavior, such as complete strangers giving you unsolicited advice; they may even reach out to touch your belly as if it were public property. But the annoyance of strangers groping you might be balanced by the unsolicited blessings you will also receive from strangers. Another significant aspect of the second trimester is prenatal diagnostic testing. Much of this chapter is about the different forms of prenatal testing and navigating your way medically and spiritually through this process.

Quickening

The following symptoms are listed as perfectly normal and experienced by many women during pregnancy: bleeding gums, breathlessness, constipation, muscle cramps, feeling faint, frequent urination, heartburn, morning sickness, hemorrhoids, difficulty sleeping, stretch marks, sweating, swollen ankles and fingers, yeast infections, and varicose veins. It is just not easy being pregnant. Your body begins to expand and do all sorts of other things it has never done before. As you face these challenges, you might find yourself asking the same question that Rebekah asked of herself in the Torah, "If this is so, why am I?" (Genesis 25:22). In other words, if pregnancy is supposed to be such a good thing, then why do I have to suffer like this?

But then it happens. You feel a little fluttering, a little something that could be mistaken for gas bubbles. You think you know what just happened, but you are not sure because it was so subtle. But then it happens again and it is undeniable; you have felt your child move for the first time. Sometime between sixteen and twenty weeks of pregnancy, you will have your first sensation of fetal movement. This is referred to as quickening.

Quickening is a small step on the road to birth. There are no traditional Jewish rituals or prayers that acknowledge it, and yet it is a profound moment. It is the concrete recognition that a potential someone is growing. Life is going on inside you.

This blessing is taken from the morning liturgy. We suggest that you sit for a moment, quietly drinking in the knowledge of movement; when you are ready, pray the following:

Prayer Following Quickening

בָּרוּךְ אַתָּה יְיָ אֲשֶׁר בְּיָדוֹ נֶפֶשׁ כָּל־חַי וְרוּחַ כָּל־בָּשָׂר.

Barukh atah Adonai asher biyado nefesh kol chai v'ruach kol basar.

Blessed are You, Adonai, in whose hand is the breath of all life and the spirit of all flesh.

Will My Child Be Normal?

As a prospective parent, you probably wonder every day about how your child will look, about her or his personality, but most importantly you wonder, "Will my child be normal?" There are a number of tests that can be done late in the first trimester and during the second trimester to screen the fetus for abnormalities. Diagnostic testing can lead to some difficult decisions. In this section, we review the tests that are currently available and provide the perspective of Jewish law as well as spiritual support to aid you as you move through this process.

Prenatal diagnostic testing is a relatively recent development. As a result of modern medical research, you can now find out whether you are at risk for carrying a baby with Tay-Sachs disease or whether your baby has Down's syndrome. In the old days, everyone took what they got, but now we have choices. You may consider these choices to be a blessing or a curse. Sandy often tells her patients that we are in an imperfect era of testing. There are an array of tests, but some tests give uncertain answers and others, such as amniocentesis, give certain answers but may pose a risk to the pregnancy.

It is important to remember that it is your choice whether to do prenatal diagnostic testing. Before taking any test, we suggest that you and your partner discuss what you will do with the information each test will provide. If a screening test indicates that there may be a problem, will you want to do a follow-up test, such as amniocentesis? If the test shows that your child has a disease such as Down's syndrome, will you terminate the pregnancy? (See the section below on Jewish perspectives on abortion.) Are you unsure about what you will do, but feel that you would like to know, at least to prepare yourself? On the other hand, does the risk of miscarriage as a result of a test seem worse to you than the possibility that your child may have a problem?

These are difficult questions. We encourage you to speak candidly with each other and think deeply about these possibilities before you take any test. If you have certain risk factors for having a child with an abnormality, such as a family history of a problem, or if you will be thirty-five or older when the baby is born, you may have to consider these questions even more seriously. And the decision may feel even more complicated if you had trouble getting pregnant. It may be helpful to discuss testing with your obstetrician, your midwife, or a genetic counselor.

We offer this *kavvana* (intention) for making your way through this process:

Kavvana for a Healthy Child

May God, the spirit of the world, our partner in creating this pregnancy, give us strength and help us now to choose the right path. We ask you, Compassionate One, for a healthy child.

Prenatal Diagnostic Testing

We've provided information here to help you understand how prenatal diagnostic testing works. This is a brief explanation of each of the tests available as of this writing. The technology for these tests is constantly improving, so please check with your obstetrician or midwife for updates. Some of the tests are blood tests, usually of the pregnant woman, but genetic tests may need to be done on the father of the baby as well. Other tests are invasive, such as an amniocentesis, which involves using a needle to withdraw amniotic fluid.

Blood tests: genetic testing

There are specific diseases that disproportionately affect Ashkenazi Jews (Jews of Eastern European origin). Genetic testing will enable you and your partner to discover whether you carry the genes for these diseases. You may choose to be tested for these before you try to conceive or after you are already pregnant. At this time, there are no specific genetic tests for the Sephardic population (Jews of Spanish, Portuguese, Turkish, and North African descent).

Briefly, genes are the blueprint for the development of humans and other living things. We are made up of cells, and in each cell there are countless numbers of genes that tell the cell what kind of cell to be and what to do (and no, we have not identified a gene that tells a Jewish child to become a doctor). The genes are organized into rodlike collections called chromosomes. Humans have twenty-three pairs of chromosomes, for a total of forty-six.

Chromosomal abnormalities refer to the absence or duplication of all or part of a chromosome. For example, Down's syndrome is a duplication of chromosome 21. Genetic diseases may be caused by either a single gene or multiple genes. A disease may be *dominant*; that is, receiving a single copy of the gene from either parent means that the child will have the disease. If one parent has a dominant gene, the child will have a 50-percent chance of being born with the disease. A disease may be *recessive*; that is, a child must receive a gene from each parent to acquire the disease. If a person has one copy of a recessive gene, he or she is called a *carrier*. If both parents are carriers of a recessive gene, their child has a 25-percent chance of being born with the disease.

The American College of Obstetricians and Gynecologists recommends screening Ashkenazi Jews for three genetic diseases: cystic fibrosis, Tay-Sachs disease, and Canavan disease. You may also be offered testing for other diseases. For complete information on diseases that affect the Jewish population, please consult the website for the National Foundation for Jewish Genetic Diseases: www.nfjgd.org.

- Cystic fibrosis (CF) is a recessive mutation; one in twenty-nine Ashkenazi Jews are CF carriers.[2] The disease is a chronic, progressive disorder that primarily affects the lungs and gastrointestinal systems. The average life expectancy for a person with CF is thirty years.

◆ Tay-Sachs disease is a recessive mutation; one in thirty Ashkenazi Jews are Tay-Sachs disease carriers.[3] In Tay-Sachs disease, a substance accumulates in the brain and causes cognitive and physical deterioration. The most common form is infantile Tay-Sachs, in which symptoms appear during the first four to eight months of life. Death usually occurs by age five.

◆ Canavan disease is a recessive mutation; one in forty Ashkenazi Jews are Canavan disease carriers.[4] In Canavan disease, a substance damages the nerve sheaths in the brain, causing progressive loss of cognitive and physical function. The symptoms appear in the first few months of life; most children die by age ten.

Blood tests: triple and quadruple screens, PAPP-A

Other blood tests are offered during the first and second trimesters to measure the risk of problems not specific to Ashkenazi Jews. The triple and quadruple screens, also referred to as the alpha-fetoprotein (AFP) tests, measure levels of specific substances in the pregnant woman's blood. The results are used to screen for neural tube defects, which lead to spina bifida, and to calculate a risk ratio for Down's syndrome and other chromosomal abnormalities. These tests cannot yield a definitive diagnosis. One of these tests is offered to all pregnant women, regardless of age. The tests are done between fifteen and twenty-two weeks' gestation. Whether you are offered the triple or quadruple screen depends upon the preference of your physician or midwife's practice.

A newer test to screen for Down's syndrome during the first trimester is available at some medical centers. This test is done between eleven and fourteen weeks. In this test, an ultrasound measurement is combined with blood tests to measure pregnancy-associated plasma protein A (PAPP-A) and human chorionic gonadotropin (hCG).

Ultrasound

You may have just one ultrasound or many during your pregnancy. Most pregnant women will at least have an ultrasound examination between sixteen and twenty weeks' gestation. Ultrasound can be used to ensure that the fetus does not have a heart defect or other anatomical problem. Certain ultrasound findings may raise concern about Down's syndrome or other chromosomal abnormalities. Some medical centers screen for Down's syndrome between eleven and fourteen weeks by measuring an aspect of the fetal neck, called the nuchal translucency.

For many women, undergoing an ultrasound can cause a great deal of anxiety, especially for those with a history of miscarriage or those who have had difficulty getting pregnant. The ultrasound also holds the beautiful prospect of a visual confirmation that you are really pregnant, that there is a human being growing inside you.

The following prayer, written by Rabbi Susan Silverman, can be said the morning of the ultrasound or on the days preceding the ultrasound. Try to find a moment of quiet and allow yourself to focus on the words of the prayer.

Prayer Before an Ultrasound

My God,
As life grows within me,
I hear the miraculous heartbeat
and sense stretching arms and legs
(does this emerging life sense me, as I sense You? reach to me,
    as I reach to You?)
As I hope for this tiny one's well-being
and know its vulnerability
And look upon this person-in-process

May I become closer to You,
Trusting in You, reaching for You, and seeking to live in Your
    presence.

You provide for our well-being.
In Your image, I seek my child's well-being.

You are *Av Harachaman,* Compassionate Parent,
In Your image, I seek to provide gentleness, love, and
    acceptance.

Show me
Through Your abundant goodness
The way to a holy relationship.

—Susan Silverman

Direct fetal testing

If any of the screening tests listed above indicates that your baby is at an increased risk of having a problem, you will be offered a direct fetal test. Direct tests are also offered to a woman if she will be thirty-five or older when her baby is born. Because of the cumulative risk to more than one fetus, women with multiple gestations may be offered a direct fetal test at an earlier maternal age. Direct tests involve examining actual fetal cells. These tests can therefore give a definitive answer regarding the presence of chromosomal abnormalities, such as Down's syndrome, or a specific genetic disorder, such as Tay-Sachs disease.

The most common direct test is amniocentesis, the use of a needle to remove amniotic fluid. The fluid contains fetal cells. Amniocentesis is generally performed between fifteen and eighteen weeks' gestation. The risk of miscarriage as a result of amniocentesis is one in two hundred. Some physicians offer amniocentesis between thirteen and fourteen weeks, however this may be riskier to the fetus.

There are other direct tests. Chorionic villus sampling (CVS) is available at some medical centers. CVS is a placental biopsy performed between ten and twelve weeks. It is an earlier alternative to amniocentesis, but the risk of miscarriage is higher, one in one hundred. Also, in special situations, such as when both prospective parents are carriers of a genetic disease, a couple may choose to do preimplantation genetic diagnosis (PGD). In PGD, a single cell is removed from an embryo during in vitro fertilization, allowing only healthy embryos to be placed in the uterus.

These tests can be difficult decisions and difficult experiences. You are willingly putting your fetus at risk, even if the risk is small. And the results of the tests can bring great relief or complex decisions. The following prayer gives voice to these concerns by asking God for help during this trying time:

Prayer Before an Amniocentesis

My God and God of our ancestors
You have made me in Your image.

With Your help
I, Your creation,
sought to create a new life
and You have blessed me
with one that grows within me.

My first act of courage
as a mother to this emerging being
is upon me.

Please grant the doctors wisdom and skill
and grant us all clarity in the wake of this test.

May I receive the results
—whether they bring joyful relief or painful confusion—
with the knowledge that I build my family
[with a loving partner and]
in a caring community
with whom I will celebrate joys and mourn losses.

Grant me wisdom and discernment
to make choices well
regarding this life which grows within me
ever aware of Your Loving Presence.

—Susan Silverman

What Do We Do Now?

We hope that you have made it through the testing process and have received encouraging results. The following is the prayer to be said upon receiving good news:

בָּרוּךְ אַתָּה יְיָ אֱלֹהֵינוּ מֶלֶךְ הָעוֹלָם,
הַטוֹב וְהַמֵּטִיב.

Barukh atah Adonai, eloheinu melekh ha'olam, hatov v'hameitiv.

Blessed are You, Adonai, our God, ruler of the universe, who is good and does good.

If you have received bad news, we wish you the strength to face your next step. You may have received a diagnosis of Down's syndrome or some other genetic disorder. You may have found out that your child has a heart defect or spina bifida. At a time like this, it is natural to ask of yourself, of each other, and of Judaism: "What do we do now?"

The question may arise as to whether you should continue or terminate your pregnancy. This is a heart-wrenching decision, and there are a variety of factors that will affect your choice. You may already have decided that you would not choose to end a pregnancy, no matter what. Alternatively, you may need more information to make your decision. What will it mean to raise a child with a medical condition? What will life be like for your child? Will this child have a limited life expectancy or be unable to live independently? If you have other children, what will the impact be on them? Will your child need surgery or extensive medical treatment? Do you feel that you have the emotional or financial resources to raise a child with this problem? We encourage you to speak to your doctor or midwife. She or he may be able to connect you with a pediatrician or parents' support group to help you gather more information.

Although this is ultimately a very personal decision, you are not alone. This is a time when you may need to work hard to make sure that you and your partner listen to each other fully. You will need to support each other to make a choice that both of you can live with. Remember that many pregnant women and their partners have found themselves in this situation. It may be helpful to find a support group or individuals in your community who are experiencing or have experienced similar problems.

Carrying a fetus with a problem

Several years ago, Dan's synagogue hosted a very special Bat Mitzvah. The Bat Mitzvah girl, in addition to being well-loved by everyone and a part of one of the synagogue's most involved families, has Down's syndrome. In a moving speech, the girl's mother said, "When a couple is expecting a baby, people often ask if they are hoping for a boy or a girl. The common response is, 'It doesn't matter as long as it's healthy.' And people do mean that . . . until the baby is born healthy, and then they want him or her to be at least normal, and hopefully perfect." The mother continued by affirming how much richer her life is for having had a child who is not "normal." Knowing that you are carrying a child who is potentially not "normal" brings an enormous amount of stress, but there is also the possibility for blessing.

From the perspective of thirteen years after the birth, Sandy Slavet, the mother of that child, reflects on the blessing her child has been:

> My daughter is adorable, funny, loving, whimsical, kind, spiritual. She has a loving relationship with her dad and me. She adores her sisters—as they adore her, and I am confident they will embrace the responsibility of overseeing her care someday when we no longer can. They speak often of honoring that promise. I can't speak to the quality of her life. But as I watch her each day—watch her laugh with her friends, watch her cut pictures out of magazines of her favorite TV/music stars,

watch her dream about her future—I see her dreams are as exciting and important to her as dreams are for all of us.

For parents who decide to continue to carry a fetus with a problem, we offer the following prayer. May it be a source of continuing strength for you during your pregnancy:

Prayer for Carrying a Fetus with a Problem

Praised are You, Eternal God—our God—Spirit of our world
You, who creates all life
You have taught us "it is good"

You have created this life—her life
Help me to trust enough—
to grow enough—
to love enough—
to know that this life that you have created is good—enough

Guide me to see all that is possible
to understand what is good and beautiful in Your eyes
to close my eyes to what I thought was "supposed to be"
and open my heart and soul to what is
and . . .
Give me the strength and courage to love what is

Praised are You, our God—who teaches us to see the potential
    in all life, and know it is good.

—Sandy Slavet

Aborting a fetus with a problem: Jewish perspectives

Upon receiving news of a fetus with a serious problem, some women and their partners may wish to terminate the pregnancy. The decision to have an abortion in this situation is, of course, profoundly difficult, and many parents look to Jewish tradition for guidance on this topic.

Before we discuss Jewish viewpoints on this issue, we should note that there is no single Jewish position on any question of medical ethics. There are many Jewish opinions, none of which is the final word. This may be frustrating to some who are looking for a single answer about what Jews believe, but contrasting opinions have been a hallmark of Jewish thought for thousands of years. In our discussion, we provide different Jewish perspectives from across the spectrum of Jewish life.

We have highlighted certain key opinions held by the different movements of Judaism today. Jews have been writing about the ethics of abortion for hundreds of years; a full cataloging of Jewish writing on this topic is beyond the scope of this chapter. We encourage you to use the information below as an introduction. References for deeper study are provided at the end of the book.

There is one point upon which all Jewish medical ethicists agree: If the fetus presents an immediate danger to the health of the mother, then it is not only permissible to have an abortion, it is required. The Mishnah states the process in a somewhat gruesome fashion:

> If a woman has [life-threatening] difficulty in childbirth, one dismembers the embryo in her, limb by limb, because her life takes precedence over its life. Once its head [or "its greater part"] has emerged, it may not be touched, for we do not set aside one life for another. (*Ohalot* 7:6)

This passage sets the precedent that the fetus does not have the same status as the mother, but once its head (or in the case of a breech birth, the buttocks and hips) comes into the world, then the fetus's status changes to be equal to the mother, and abortion at this point is no longer permissible.

There is also agreement that it is permissible, but not required, to have an abortion under certain circumstances if the mother's health is jeopardized but not in an immediate danger, as in the passage above. The differences in Jewish opinion occur when the question is asked, "What is the definition of a danger to the mother's health?" This has been interpreted broadly by some Jewish thinkers to include a threat to the psychological health of the mother by carrying an unwanted child. Others have interpreted this much more narrowly, permitting abortion only when the mother's physical health is in serious jeopardy.

In the case of a fetus who is found to have a problem, the differences among Jewish ethicists on the permissibility of abortion are quite stark. One of the leading Orthodox authorities on these matters, Rabbi J. David Bleich, states unequivocally that abortion based on the condition of the fetus is not permissible. He writes the following:

> Judaism regards all forms of human life as sacred, from the formation of germ plasm in the cell of the sperm until the decomposition of the body after death.... Fetal life is regarded as precious and may not be destroyed wantonly.[5]

The only concern for traditional Jewish ethicists is the mother's health. Bleich rejects the idea that a fetus should be aborted because it will be abnormal because he understands all life to be imbued with the same sanctity. He also rejects the idea that a woman might be so psychologically ill-prepared for or harmed by raising a baby with problems that her health will be endangered. Bleich is not impervious to the difficulty parents face in raising such children, but for him this is not enough of a consideration to abort a fetus. He even goes so far as to reject amniocentesis to uncover fetal abnormalities because the only medical treatment in cases such as Tay-Sachs disease would be an abortion, which is not permissible, so the amniocentesis should not even be done.[6]

Elliot Dorff, the leading Conservative Jewish thinker on these matters, takes a more liberal stance.[7] He begins by basing his argument on the ruling of a seventeenth-century *posek* (arbiter of Jewish law), Rabbi Israel Meir Mizrachi. Rabbi Mizrachi writes that if having a child will cause a woman to become mentally unstable, then abortion is permissible. Some modern Jewish ethicists have interpreted this position broadly to suggest that circumstances such as finding out that there is a problem with a child may endanger the mother's mental health and thus make abortion permissible.

Dorff also says that traditional Jewish thinkers take into account only the mother's health because, until recently, it was impossible to know anything about the health of the fetus. New medical knowledge "ought to establish the fetus's health as an independent consideration." Thus, he bases his position on the status of the fetus and its future quality of life, as well as on the mental health of the mother.

Dorff says that in cases such as Tay-Sachs disease and other degenerative conditions where the baby will die in a few years, abortion is clearly permissible. But he is not as clear on cases where the degeneration will not be apparent until the carrier reaches thirty-five or forty, such as Huntington's disease. He writes:

> I believe that abortion is not justified in that case, since the person will live an extended period of time without suffering from any of the disease's debilitating effects—indeed enough time to have children of his or her own and even participate in much of their rearing—and since there is a reasonable hope that a cure may be developed in that time. But where do we draw the line? [When the condition manifests itself at] twenty-five years? Fifteen years? And what constitutes a defect justifying abortion in the first place? Mental retardation? If so, how much? Blindness or deafness? We quickly slide into the danger of defining qualifications for a master race, with the corollary depreciation of disabled people.[8]

But, Dorff argues, making such distinctions is precisely what is necessary in the real world of ethical decisions. He tentatively suggests that for a fetus with Down's syndrome, for example, the determination of the permissibility of abortion should be based upon the woman's psychological competence to handle such a child. For some women this would be beyond their capabilities, while other women would be able to do such a thing. He suggests that this would raise other issues such as, "if most families abort 'defective children,' one wonders about the degree to which society in the long run will tolerate imperfections and provide for people who have them."[9]

The Reform movement of Judaism is the most liberal on the subject of abortion. The Reform movement says that abortion is permissible if there is physical or psychological danger to the mother, because the fetus does not have the status of a human being; abortion is therefore eliminating only potential life and not life itself. This is especially true in the first forty days of pregnancy. Traditionally, the fetus is considered to have the least status during the first forty days; the Talmud says that at this point the fetus is "simply water" (*Yevamot* 69b). If the authors of the Talmud were women who could already feel a change taking place in their bodies, they may not have called the fetus simply water, but the image does get across the idea that the Rabbis considered this stage to have almost no status. Thus, Rabbi Walter Jacob, writing for the Reform movement, says that during the initial forty days, abortion would be permitted for a wide array of factors that might cause psychological damage to the mother. After this period, abortion is still permissible, but the reasons need to justify the procedure.

Jacob notes that, "Such problems as those caused by Tay-Sachs and other degenerative or permanent conditions, which seriously endanger the life of the child and potentially the mental health of the mother, are indications for permitting an abortion."[10]

The Reform movement's position is based on a liberal reading of Jewish tradition. Although historically there have always been strict opponents of abortion in Judaism, the Reform movement notes that there have always been rabbis who have permitted abortion under circumstances that go beyond the case of danger to the mother. Rabbi W. Gunther Plaut and Dr. Mark Washovsky, writing for the Reform movement, cite the position of Rabbi Jacob Emden (1697–1776) as part of a responsum (Jewish legal opinion) on the permissibility of aborting an illegitimate fetus (a fetus conceived out of wedlock).[11] They write:

> Emden notes that even in the case of a legitimate fetus, "there is room to permit abortion for 'great need' so long as the birth process has not begun, even if the reason is not to save her

life—even if only to save her from the 'great pain' it causes her." Emden not only plainly articulates an outlook that countenances abortion for reasons less than a threat to the life of the mother, but he also points to the central *halakhic* [Jewish law] concern of the more lenient respondents: "great pain" caused to the mother.[12]

The central issue for the Reform movement is whether the pregnancy is causing "great pain" to the mother, either psychologically or physically. It is willing to be liberal about what might be considered an issue of great pain, and problems with the fetus certainly would qualify as such. Just to be clear, Rabbi Jacob and the Reform movement are not supporting abortion under these circumstances as the right thing for a woman. Rather, they are saying that for women who wish to terminate their pregnancies, abortion is a permissible act from a Jewish perspective.

If you are in the process of making this decision, we encourage you to speak with a rabbi and/or therapist as well as your obstetrician or midwife. We also encourage you to try to communicate with your partner as best as possible. This is such an intense decision that you need to be sure that the two of you are hearing each other's wishes clearly.

If you choose to abort your fetus, you have our sympathies. Even if there was little choice in the matter medically, the end of a potential life is painful. You had already been imagining a child in your life, and now there will not be one. Allow yourself the opportunity to mourn for the loss of this potential life.

Multiple Gestation

It's twins (or more)! There you are, laying on a table for your first ultrasound. If you hear this announcement, you are sure to feel your heart racing. You may have been prepared for the possibility of twins, triplets, or more if you got pregnant through fertility treatments. As a result of fertility medications, the rate of twins in the

United States has increased from 1.9 percent of births in 1980 to 2.9 percent in 2000.[13] If you did not expect twins (or more), this news can be quite a surprise.

Hearing that you are carrying more than one child can be great news if you have had difficulty starting a family until now. On the other hand, you and your partner may have decided to have just one more, in which case you might not be quite as thrilled. How do twins happen? Twins can be either dizygotic (fraternal) or monozygotic (identical). Fraternal twins occur when more than one egg is ovulated and fertilized. Fraternal twins are related to the same degree as any siblings. The chance of having fraternal twins increases with age and with fertility treatments. Identical twins occur when one egg splits into two embryos. This must happen during the first sixteen days after conception. If the split happens between the thirteenth and fifteenth day, conjoined (Siamese) twins will be the result. Identical twins are the product of a single egg and sperm and, therefore, have identical DNA. Triplets may be a combination of three fraternal siblings, or two identical and one fraternal. Quadruplets can be four fraternal, two identical and two fraternal, or two sets of identical twins... you see how the math works.

Carrying more than one child has its joys and challenges. It is not unusual for a woman carrying twins, and certainly triplets or more, to be on extended bed rest because of the difficulty of the pregnancy. Multiple gestations are more prone to pregnancy loss, preterm labor, and preeclampsia (see p. 61).

Long before the recent rise in the number of twins, the Torah spoke of two different sets of twins, both crucial to the biblical narrative. Each set of twins in the Torah has an unusual birthing story.

The more well-known story is Rebekah's pregnancy with Jacob and Esau, whom the Torah describes as struggling even in the womb (Genesis 25:22). The biblical Rebekah did not have that pregnancy glow; she was carrying twins and she was uncomfortable. A midrash says that Rebekah was being crushed by the pain of carrying the twins, and she went to seek advice from the other women in her community:

"Did you ever experience anything like this in your pregnancies?"

"No," they replied.

"My pains are so great," Rebekah complained, "that I wish I had never become pregnant" (*Genesis Rabbah* 63:6).

When the day of their birth finally arrives, Esau is born first, with Jacob holding his heel. (Jacob's name in Hebrew, *Yaakov*, literally means "heel"). From a medical perspective, the birth of Jacob and Esau is quite interesting if we take the Torah literally. Is it possible for twins to come out holding on to each other? Yes, but only if they are identical and share an amniotic sac or if both sacs were broken before delivery.

The relationship of Jacob and Esau forms a central part of the Genesis narrative. The struggling in the womb only becomes worse when they get outside of it. Jacob famously steals the blessing of the firstborn from his brother Esau, by dressing up as Esau to fool their blind father. Esau's response is to want to kill Jacob, which sends Jacob fleeing from home for years. After Jacob marries (twice, not to mention two concubines) and has twelve kids, he goes back home to see his brother in what is surely one of the most climactic moments in the Torah. Jacob falls down before his brother seven times asking for forgiveness. They dramatically run toward each other and embrace, letting the years of enmity fall away.

The Torah suggests something about the psychological connection between twins. Even in the womb Jacob and Esau struggled with each other; their lives were destined to have conflict with each other. But the connection between the two also suggests that they could not live without each other. They were incomplete until they resolved their differences. After Jacob and Esau make up, the text says that "Jacob came *complete* to the city of Shechem" (Genesis 33:18). What does the word "complete" mean in this situation? It might mean that Jacob came unharmed to the city, but another interpretation is that Jacob was now, after having embraced his twin brother, complete. Even after many years and many life events, Jacob's unresolved relationship with his twin was a driving force in his life. Such is the power, the Torah seems to be saying, of two beings born from the same womb at the same time.

The lesser-known story involves Tamar's twins, Peretz and Zerach. Tamar has a sexual encounter with her father-in-law, Judah, after the death of her two husbands, both of whom were Judah's sons (Genesis 38). As Peretz is being born, he sticks out an arm on which the midwife places a scarlet thread. However, the arm then goes back into the womb, and his brother Zerach is born first, followed by Peretz and his scarlet thread.

In both these stories of twins—Jacob and Esau and Peretz and Zerach—the primary concern of the Bible seems to be who is born first. The firstborn is the successor to the head of the house, the one who passes along the family line, and the one who inherits the property. The Torah also says that the firstborn son is sacred, the exclusive possession of God. The custom of *pidyon haben*, the redemption of the firstborn, comes from this understanding. *Pidyon haben* is a ceremony performed thirty days after the birth of the firstborn son of the mother.[14] The ceremony involves "buying" back the child from God via a *kohain* (a person of Jewish priestly lineage), usually for five silver coins.

In the Torah, both these stories of twins are cases of the natural order being overturned and the younger son becoming the important one in carrying on the family line. Jacob, of course, becomes a patriarch of the Jewish people. Peretz is named in the lineage of King David. The Torah was obviously fascinated with twins and the implicit symbolism of two who are so intimately connected. We hope for you that twins do not bring the strife and pain they caused Rebekah, but only double the joy of motherhood.

Selective Reduction: Jewish Perspectives

Fertility treatments have greatly increased the number of twins, triplets, quadruplets, and even quintuplets in the world. Some women, particularly those who used fertility treatments, may find themselves carrying two or more fertilized eggs and considering selective reduction. Selective reduction refers to terminating one or more of the fetuses while not harming the other fetuses.

We discussed Jewish views on abortion in general in a previous section and, as we noted there, the health of the mother is of paramount importance. If the mother's health is endangered by multiple gestation, selective abortion is permissible. Elliot Dorff writes that if genetic testing could show which of the fetuses would be least likely to survive, it would be permissible to abort that particular fetus(es); if, however, all the fetuses are equally viable, then the reduction should be done randomly.[15]

Some Orthodox authorities have taken the position that if a woman is carrying more than three fertilized embryos, she can selectively reduce the number down to three because carrying more than three fetuses would by definition pose great harm to the mother's mental and physical health. However, if a woman is carrying three fetuses and would like to reduce down to twins out of an unwillingness to have three children at once, traditional authorities would say this was not permissible. Liberal Jewish ethicists have not yet officially addressed this issue.

Sephardic Celebration of Pregnancy

Having spent much of this chapter discussing potential difficulties, we would like to end the chapter on a note of joy. We mentioned earlier that Judaism is hesitant about celebrating pregnancy, knowing that not all pregnancies end with a healthy baby. Therefore, most Jewish celebrations are put off until the baby is born. Some Sephardic Jews, however, have a celebration to mark the second trimester of pregnancy. In *A Time to Be Born*, Michelle Klein describes one such celebration by Jews in Istanbul that is still in practice today. The celebration entails making the first cuts into a cloth that will become the baby's first clothing. If you are inclined to take the Sephardic approach, we provide the following description of this custom to inspire you. The ceremony is called *kortadura de fashadura* in Ladino,[16] meaning "the cutting of the swaddling clothes."

Klein describes the ceremony as follows:

The ceremonial cutting of a cloth to make the baby's first costume, which is the same for a boy or a girl, is an old Sephardic custom still continued by some Jews in Istanbul. When a Jewish woman reaches her fifth month of her first pregnancy,[17] her family invites all her female relatives and in-laws, as well as friends and neighbors. Liquors and chocolates, tea, cakes, and sugared almonds are set out on the best china, on hand-embroidered tablecloths. . . . A relative who is herself a mother and whose parents are still alive (a good omen for a long life) receives the honors of making the first cut in the cloth. At the moment of the cut, the pregnant woman throws white sugared almonds on the cloth, to symbolize the sweet and prosperous future she wishes for her child.[18]

3
___

The Third Trimester

Y ou have come to the third and final trimester. Your belly is swelling and so are your ankles. The numerous complaints of Sandy's patients in the third trimester often prompt her to quip, "Isn't pregnancy glamorous?" At this point you feel strong kicks and your partner can feel them, too. You start to believe that this long, strange trip may actually produce a baby. You find yourself caught up more and more in imagining the birth of your child. This chapter will review some of the things that happen during the third trimester and the preparation process for birth.

Prayers for the Third Trimester

We prayed a lot in the third trimester. The acute anticipation of a delivery and a baby naturally brought forth some pleas to the One Who Creates Life. Following is a brief sample of prayers said in the final trimester of pregnancy.

Prayer for entering the seventh month of pregnancy
When you enter the third trimester you may start counting down the days until your due date. The third trimester is God's lesson in patience and perseverance. The following prayer is said when a women enters the seventh month of pregnancy; it emphasizes the idea that the baby should be born at the appropriate hour, whenever

that hour may be. The prayer is adapted from an eighteenth-century Italian prayer book for women:

> Lord our God and God of our forebears, may it be Your will that I easily suffer the strains of pregnancy. Continually grant me stamina throughout the pregnancy so that the baby's strength may not fail, nor mine, in any way. Let the child be born speedily, and may I give birth easily and quickly without any harm either to me or to the child. Let the child be born when the time is right, at a propitious moment, so he may enjoy a full life of peace, health, and pleasantness, of goodness, prosperity and honor.[1]

Prayer said by a partner

For the partner of a pregnant woman, one of the most difficult parts of pregnancy is knowing that your loved one will be in some pain during labor and knowing that there is nothing you can do about it. Yes, you have tried to be supportive when she had morning sickness, when she had cravings, and when she couldn't put on her shoes. You will be supportive during the delivery, but you are helpless to take away the pain.

Praying for an easy delivery for a partner is a traditional part of Judaism. The Talmud records that during the first trimester the husband should pray that his wife will not miscarry; during the second trimester he should pray that the baby will not be stillborn; and during the third trimester he should pray for a safe delivery (*Berakhot* 60a). Initially, these prayers were private, spontaneous prayers, but around the seventeenth century they were written down. The following is an edited version of a prayer first published in the mid-nineteenth century in a prayer book called *Beit Tefillah* (House of Prayer) by Eleazer Papo:

> God, I thank You for your kindness, for helping my wife become pregnant with our child.
>
> God, may it be your will to show kindness to all pregnant women and ease the discomforts of their pregnancies. Pro-

tect them so that none of them miscarries. Guard all who are in the throes of labor, so that no harm comes to them and that they give birth to life. Include among them my wife [her name]. Ease her pain, lighten her burden, let her complete the months of pregnancy and give birth with ease. Let no mar or blemish or illness come upon my wife or the child. Let our little one be fully formed with all physical and mental capacities. *El Harachaman,* God of mercy, deal with us mercifully, and not according to the laws of strict justice. Overlook our weaknesses and misdeeds, and act towards us with kindness and graciousness. Give us long life, and let my wife and me grow old together, proud of our children, watching them do your will.[2]

Prayer for a good neshama (soul)

The following passage is from Martha Hausman, who reflects on praying for her child as she entered the last trimester:

> The Mishnah teaches: "One who prays for something that has already happened is making a false prayer." The first example given is, "A man whose wife is pregnant, and prays, 'May she give birth to a boy,' has made a false prayer [because the sex of the child has already been determined at the moment of conception]" (*Berakhot* 9:3).
>
> When I was pregnant, I wanted to talk to God about the baby more than I had ever wanted to talk to God before, but inside I knew that I could not ask God to change anything that had already been decided. And, as we know so much about science these days, I knew that from conception all the chromosomes had been chosen, the gene combinations assigned. Still, my need to pray for it was strong.
>
> I am not a huge personal pray-er. But when I was pregnant I needed to express myself more. The baby inside me seemed inextricably linked to God. It felt as if the baby *was* God's; I had just been selected to carry and, eventually, to take care of it. Although this concept is part of Jewish tradition, I wasn't thinking about that. It was a natural and insistent feeling. God was still making this baby, but how could I participate? What could I ask God for?

I prayed for the baby's soul. Its *neshama*, that which would make the child—the person—essentially who he or she would be. I was praying for its presence—the way a room would change when he or she walked into it, my child's effect on his or her world, as well as my child's sense of self. Tears came. Not once, but time after time during the pregnancy. Please, God, a beautiful soul. Choose a compassionate one, a loving one. Make it funny. And serious. I promise to nurture the qualities you bestow. To do everything I can to help my child be a blessing and a light to the world.

—Martha Hausman

B'sha-ah Tovah: Jewish Customs When It Comes to Baby Showers

It is common in the third trimester for women to be given a baby shower by friends and relatives, who shower her with baby clothes and items for the baby's room. When Sandy was pregnant, people often asked her, "Is the baby's room ready?" She would say, "Yes . . . it is completely empty." According to Jewish custom, one does *not* furnish a baby room in any way. It is also Jewish custom *not* to have a baby shower. This surprises some people, Jews included, who are expecting to get some of the baby goods lined up before the big day. But Judaism understands that the baby needs to arrive first before getting the stuff. The cautious Jewish attitude continues throughout the pregnancy. Judaism respects the mystery and danger that are still part of pregnancy today. You are still in the *b'sha-ah tovah* phase; that is, you are still in the phase where birth is still potential. You only get to *mazel tov*, congratulations, when the baby is born. Apparently, there are other cultures that share this viewpoint. We have friends who say that their old Irish aunts shudder when they see baby gifts around the house before the birth.

The purpose of this practice is to protect you emotionally, just in case, God forbid, something goes wrong with the delivery and you don't return home with a baby. Seeing a room full of baby things could only add to what would already be an incredibly difficult experience. Practically, you'll be fine if you hold off on buying things. A new baby just needs a bassinet in which to sleep, a few pieces of clothing, and a few diapers (well, okay, a lot of diapers). (Just between you and us, many people deal with this custom by putting things on order and storing things somewhere outside the house.)

Your family, friends, and coworkers may nag you about throwing you a shower. You can let them show their love for you with a slightly alternative, mother-focused event. Sandy had a birth support party with a group of close friends. They shared their own birth stories and gave her their blessings, and they prepared a book for her to take to the hospital.

The following is a ritual written by Rabbi Shohama Wiener that we have adapted to use at a birth support party.

A birthing support ritual: blessings for a mother-to-be

Seating: Seat six close friends or relatives around the mother-to-be in the form of a six-pointed *magen david*, star of protection and blessing. Everyone else should sit in concentric circles extending out. If it is not possible to sit in this form, seat the mother-to-be at the head of a circle.

Opening *niggun* (wordless melody).

Blessings

[Ask the group to say "Amen" after each blessing.]

Makor Hachayyim v'Rofeh Hacholim, Source of Life and Divine Healer, give blessing and health, safety and ease of childbirth to [name of mother], and to her baby who yet grows within.

May the little one emerge at a *b'sha-ah tovah*, a goodly hour, an hour of ripeness and readiness for entering this world in health and in joy.

May [parent's name] and [parent's name] grow ever closer as they prepare for the blessed experience of becoming parents.

May [name of mother] remain healthy, joyful, and strong as she prepares to be a Mother-in-Israel.

And may all [mother's name]'s circle of loved ones keep her in their hearts and prayers during this precious time of anticipation.

May our prayers be signed and sealed. Let us all say, Amen.

[Name of mother], I give to you a red thread symbolic of the red threads from the place where our biblical mother Rachel dwells, called *Kever Rachel,* Rachel's Tomb.[3] This thread holds the prayers of many pious women, prayers for health and safety during pregnancy and delivery. Keep it near you.

We also have a cup of water that holds our blessings for you.

[Each participant holds the cup, says a personal blessing for the mother-to-be, and rubs a few drops on the hands of the mother-to-be.]

[The mother-to-be may offer a blessing for the fetus she carries.]

Closing *niggun* and dance.

Preparing to Become a Jewish Parent

As you have reached the final trimester, your thoughts are focusing more and more not only on the delivery, but also on the actual being that is going to emerge from you and what it will mean to be a parent. The following essay from Joanna Selznick Dulkin is a reflection on what it means to be a Jewish parent, and it offers some basic wisdom for nurturing a Jewish soul.

Between prenatal care visits, buying new clothes for your expanding body, and gaining wisdom from friends and family, you should also take time to reflect on your new role as a Jewish parent. You now have the unique opportunity to become a part of a sacred tradition of parents and children.

Jewish tradition enumerates several distinct responsibilities of parents to children.

+ To provide ethical and moral teaching in accordance with Jewish tradition. We pass on the teachings of who we are as a living, breathing Torah. What is the Torah you wish to pass on to your children, and how will it manifest itself throughout your lifetime and theirs?

+ To set and maintain boundaries of acceptable behavior. We have a code of *mitzvot:* commandments that set boundaries for Jewish behavior. How are you going to create a nurturing, loving Jewish home? Think about how you will ritually welcome this child into the Jewish community, and how this welcoming ritual will set the stage for your child's relationship to Judaism and to *mitzvot*. What are some commitments you will strive to make to create an atmosphere for growth and learning? How will you use Jewish values to set clear boundaries and reinforce them?

+ To provide material, emotional, and spiritual support. Providing for our children not only means setting aside money for tuition, health care, clothing, and allowance, it also means supporting them emotionally. Keep in touch with your children's emotional and social development as well as their physical and academic development, and be there when they need you. Honor their spiritual searching, answer questions as honestly as you can, helping them find the answer if you don't have it. Don't teach anything you'll have to eventually un-teach, and know that you are an exemplar in what you do as much as in what you say.

+ To provide blessing. Judaism has a powerful tradition of parents blessing their children that continues to this day. On Friday nights, Jewish parents across the world bless their children at the Shabbat dinner table, saying, "May you be like Ephraim and Menasseh," to boys and "May you be like Sarah, Rebekah, Rachel, and Leah," to girls, then offering their children the holy words of the priestly blessing, "May God bless you and keep you. May God's light shine upon you and be gracious to you. May God lift God's face towards you and grant you peace."

According to the Talmud, a father has certain obligations to his son (*Kiddushin* 30b). The father must circumcise his son, perform *pidyon haben* (see page 38), teach him Torah, betroth him to a woman, teach him a trade, and some authorities say he must teach him to swim. The father's obligations to his daughter include providing her with clothing, and giving her a dowry up to one-tenth of his wealth (so that men may be anxious to woo her and marry her).

Some of the obligations of a father still seem meaningful today, such as teaching Torah and Jewish values to your child. I would, however, interpret some of these obligations in a slightly different way than the Rabbis had in mind, and I would expand them to include mothers as well as fathers.

Because today the majority of parents no longer choose their children's spouses (as much as they might want to), I would suggest that "betrothing him to a woman" be reinterpreted as the parental responsibility to model healthy relationships; to instill in their children the self-esteem and compassion for others to enable them to find a partner and sustain a relationship.

A contemporary reworking of the list of talmudic obligations could read: "Parents are obligated to bring their children into the covenant through a public ritual; provide them with clothing and shelter; teach them Torah; teach them to read; counsel them towards higher education and employment; teach them that their job is not only what they do during work but their job is also to make the world a better place; foster their self-esteem, and some say teach them to swim."

Why swim? "Because [the child's] life might depend on it," the Talmud answers. Swimming is the defense against drowning: it is up to parents to equip the children with skills so that they can make choices and act to, as our tradition says, "choose life." A swimming lesson becomes a life lesson. Teaching our children to swim today is about teaching them to say no to a cigarette, or how to stay cool while not doing drugs or driving drunk; teaching them how to defend themselves on a dark street. In teaching our children these things, we are in effect teaching them how to choose life, one of the most important *mitzvot* of all.

—Joanna Selznick Dulkin

Preparing for Birth

As the end of your pregnancy approaches, you will be making final decisions and preparations for the birth. These may include choosing who will be with you for the big event, what you will bring with you, and whether you plan to have anesthesia for delivery. These questions are primarily predicated on your having a baby in the hospital, and may not apply for those who choose home births. At the end of this section we provide a brief guide for those thinking about home births.

What should you bring? A Jewish packing list

For many expectant couples who plan to give birth in the hospital, packing "the bag" becomes a focal point for the anxiety of the approaching birth. We dealt with this by just leaving a bag open and throwing things into it as we thought of them. Of course, be sure to bring your camera, a change of underwear and socks, and one outfit for the baby; if you forget anything else, don't worry, you'll be fine.

To go along with the clothes and the camera, we would like to suggest a Jewish packing list. First on the Jewish packing list are objects that will make your delivery room feel spiritually like your own space. We suggest that you imagine your delivery room as your tent. This particular image derives from Jewish tradition. A midrash says that there are angels who are charged with guarding a woman as she labors. These angels are called by the name *yitadot*, literally "tent pegs."[4] Tent pegs are a rich symbol in Jewish tradition. At a basic level, they suggest you are securing a temporary dwelling. You are placing tent pegs to transform a space into a home for yourself, a *sukat shalom*, a refuge of peace.

Tent pegs in the Jewish imagination are also associated with the biblical story of Yael, from the Book of Judges. The story of Yael takes place during a war between the Israelites and the Canaanites. Led by Deborah the judge, the Israelites destroyed the Canaanite army in a battle, and the leader of the Canaanites, Sisera, fled. Yael, the wife of Heber, welcomed Sisera into her tent under the pretext of helping him, though she was secretly plotting to kill him. Yael told Sisera to lie down and rest. While he was sleeping, she took a tent peg and smashed it through his skull. Yael, like Deborah, the other heroine in the story, is a rare biblical figure of female strength.[5]

Tent pegs are thus a symbol of temporary security as well as raw female strength, and you will need both of these as you deliver. We suggest symbolically setting up your delivery room as your tent; one way to do so is to place four objects in the corners of your room as you arrive. These four items may be personal items that make the room feel like your own, or you could go further with the symbolism and bring items representing your past, your present, your future, and your hope for the baby. You could bring items representing peace and strength. There are any number of ways to construct your tent.

Bringing a symbolic physical presence into the delivery room is apparently not a unique idea. A colleague of Sandy's once told her the following story. After the baby was born, the couple started to giggle. The obstetrician asked what was so funny, and the wife said, "Okay, since you are from Texas, I guess we can tell you. Everyone in both our families as far as the mind can recall has been born on Texas soil. We felt that this child should be no exception." At that point the father reached under the bed, which was located in Boston, Massachusetts. He pulled out a bag of dirt, and said "We brought this from Texas, especially for the birth."

Another item on the Jewish packing list is a focal point. Many women, whether they are giving birth with or without anesthesia, bring in a visual item to help them concentrate while they push. Women who have had a previous child sometimes bring a picture of the first child. As a Jewish focal point, you may want to bring a *shviti*. A *shviti* is a traditional Jewish art form used for meditation. *Shvitis* do not all look exactly alike, but they all have a verse from the Book of Psalms, "I have set God always before me" (Psalms 16:8), placed in a picture that is meant to encourage a meditative state. *Shvitis* are available in Judaica shops, and with a little effort can be found in a variety of places online. See page 52 for an example of a contemporary *shviti*.

Other items to consider for a Jewish packing list are a *siddur* (prayer book) or the Book of Psalms. You may want to bring this book you are reading right now with you or copy the prayers that you find most meaningful to have on hand. Finally, consider bringing music and a CD player with you. We suggest the following CDs as possibilities: *Tuning the Soul*, by Richard Kaplan and Michael Ziegler; *With Every Breath*, by Congregation B'nai Jeshurun; and *Enchant-meant*, by Shefa Gold.

We should note that in the next chapter we provide a number of brief *kavvanot* (intentions) for labor and delivery. You may want to do a little bit of preparation and memorize one of these to be ready for labor. As labor progresses, you will be unable to read, of course, so having some mantra that you can repeat over and over as a focus will offer you spiritual support.

Who will accompany you?

You may have chosen either a midwife or an obstetrician to handle your labor and delivery. Some women also choose to have a *doula*, a professional labor support person. If you are approaching labor alone or with a partner who gets queasy when things start to get messy, we suggest that you seriously consider hiring a *doula*. Certainly consider it if you are thinking of natural childbirth, and perhaps even if you are planning on having an epidural. It is helpful to have someone really focused on you and your needs throughout the

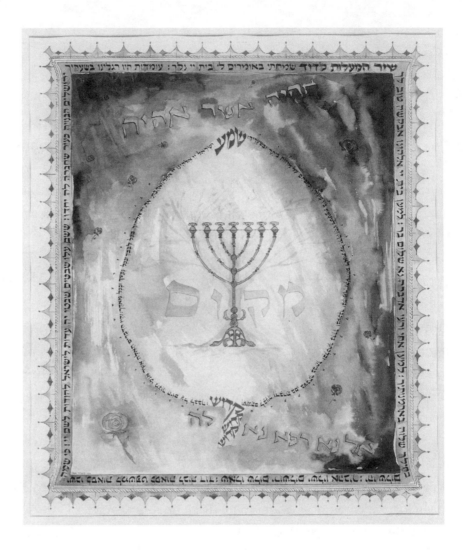

Spiritual Symbolism. In the center of the *shviti* pictured above, you see the menorah; the Tree of Life is in the background. Surrounding the menorah and Tree of Life is an *etrog*, the symbol of fertility and joy associated with Sukkot. The edge of the *etrog* is the *Sh'ma* and the *v'ahavta,* Judaism's most well-known prayers, which ask each of us to love God with all our heart and soul. Above each word of the *v'ahavta* is a small letter. The forty-two words of the *v'ahavta* correspond to a mystical name of God, which is forty-two letters long. Below the *etrog* is the shortest prayer in the Torah, which Moses says on behalf of his sister Miriam, *"El na refa na la!"* "God please heal her now!" (Numbers 12:13). There are ten roses scattered around the *etrog,* one for each of the *sefirot*. The psalm around the edge is Psalm 122. This is the psalm of arrival and happiness.

process. In addition to your birth attendant and your partner, this is a good time to consider whether you also wish to invite a friend or family member to be there for your labor and delivery.

Think of labor as a marathon. Marathon runners will often tell their friends to wait for them at exactly the seventeenth or nineteenth mile, whatever point they think they will need the most encouragement. (We have a friend who has run marathons and given birth and she says that there is simply no question which is harder—she'll take the twenty-six mile run any day. "At least running you can stop if you absolutely have to.")

This is a good time to talk with your labor partner about how he/she will be helpful to you. There are many ways your partner can assist you: massaging you, helping you with focused breathing, getting you ice chips, helping you into a different position, or just saying encouraging things like, "You're doing great." It may sound silly, but we definitely suggest that you consider ahead of time what specific encouraging words you want your partner to say to you when the times comes.

Drugs or not?

One of the questions you need to address ahead of time is whether you will take pain medication during delivery. We considered titling this book *The Jewish Pregnancy Book: Oy, Where Is My Epidural?* but thought better of it.

In the first half of the twentieth century, labor pain was commonly treated with morphine and scopolamine, causing women to be quite drowsy and, often, unable to even remember the delivery.[6] This method was called "twilight sleep" and was thought to be a compassionate way of saving women from the pain of childbirth. Women's rebellion against this treatment led to the "natural childbirth" movement. If you choose natural childbirth, that is, to deliver without any pain medication, you may wish to take a class to prepare yourself. There are several approaches, including Lamaze, the Bradley method, and hypnobirthing. Lamaze is the most well known and focuses on breathing as a way of coping with the pain during delivery. A basic birthing class is offered in many hospitals and would be good to take regardless of whether or not you are going to have an epidural.

Currently, an epidural is the most common type of obstetrical anesthesia. An epidural is called a regional anesthetic. It provides pain relief to an entire region of the body—in this case, from the waist down. It works like this: a catheter is placed in your lower back to deliver pain medication to the layer of fat around your spinal cord, which is called the epidural space. A functioning epidural will relieve the pain of contractions and much of the pain of delivery. You will still need to push to deliver the child. Epidurals, like so much in medicine, have improved in recent years; they now can numb much of the pain, but they do not reduce all feeling, so you will still be able to feel the contractions. The major question most woman have is whether using an epidural has any ill effects for the baby. Epidurals are considered safe for your baby.

There is no Jewish position on using drugs such as an epidural during labor. There is nothing written in Jewish tradition about natural childbirth, nor is there any standard belief about the value of pain. Natural childbirth is ultimately a personal choice about how you want your labor experience to be.

Home Birthing

Throughout our long, rich history, Jewish women have given birth in tents, in fields, and at home. Some women still choose to give birth at home. You may be interested in giving birth at home if you feel that this can offer you a warmer, more holistic experience than you would have in a hospital. Deciding whether to have a home birth comes down to weighing risks. Most deliveries will go fine without a high level of medical intervention. However, when something goes wrong, it can go wrong quickly, putting mother and baby in danger. One example of such an emergency is a prolapse of the umbilical cord. In such a situation, the baby's umbilical cord emerges from the cervix before the baby's head. The cord is then compressed by the head, cutting off the baby's blood supply. The only way to save the baby is to deliver the baby by emergency C-section within minutes of the prolapse.

If you are thinking about having a home birth, we encourage you to make careful preparations. Choose your midwife carefully, and check her qualifications and record. Make sure that your midwife has an official relationship with an obstetrician and a hospital, and speak with that obstetrician at some point during your pregnancy. If you know that your pregnancy poses risks, it may be wiser not to plan a home birth. Also, make sure that during your pregnancy you are tested for common complications of pregnancy, including gestational diabetes and preeclampsia. Finally, if you find yourself attracted to birthing outside a hospital setting but are not comfortable with home birthing, a birthing center, if there is one in your area, may be a nice compromise for you.

Visiting the *Mikvah*

The *mikvah* is a Jewish ritual purification bath in which people immerse themselves completely in water (think baptism if you are totally unfamiliar with the concept). Generally, *mikvaot* (plural) are housed in small buildings, are often attached to synagogues, and consist of some changing rooms leading to a room with seven steps descending to a pool of water about four feet deep. The waters of the *mikvah* are a combination of natural rainwater and tap water. Oceans and rivers, however, constitute natural *mikvaot*.

Traditionally, using the *mikvah* is primarily a female ritual. A Jewish woman goes to the *mikvah* before her wedding, after each menstruation as a married woman, and after giving birth. Men and women who are converting to Judaism use the *mikvah* as the last step in their conversion. Recently, Jewish women have begun using the *mikvah* for alternative reasons, often seeking the healing environment of the *mikvah* waters after difficult experiences, such as completing chemotherapy, going through a divorce, or having an abortion.

In Judaism, there is also a strong association between pregnancy and using the *mikvah*. There are some stories of Chasidic women who have difficulty getting pregnant using the *mikvah* after a famous rebbe has used the *mikvah*, hoping the waters that have touched the rebbe are especially blessed and will enhance their fertility. Jewish women of all denominations have also recently taken to using the *mikvah* as a spiritual support if they are struggling with infertility.

There is a custom of women using the *mikvah* during the ninth month of pregnancy to prepare spiritually for labor and delivery. Jewish custom also holds that pregnant women have a special ability to bless others, so pregnant women in the *mikvah* may pray for others who wish to become pregnant. One custom for women who wish to become pregnant is to immerse themselves in the *mikvah* after a pregnant woman.

The following essay by Amy Friedman describes her journey to the *mikvah* when she was nine months pregnant and the blessings she encountered there. Amy also visited the *mikvah* extensively when she was trying to get pregnant. The essay is written as a journal to her child.

> During the time that we were longing for you with our full hearts, I had discovered that there is a special ritual that occurs with *mikvah* and fertility. A woman in her ninth month may immerse in the *mikvah* and pray for others. Having used the *mikvah* as a spiritual support during the long process of trying to get pregnant, I felt close to the women who wish for children. So participating in this ritual felt important to me. I was so grateful to God, and I wished to immerse not just to thank God for you, but to pray for others with any compelling power and blessing my special status as a pregnant woman might bring.
>
> On the day I went to immerse, I was exactly thirty-eight weeks, and finally I felt ready for the next stage to occur. I had

just finished tying up all loose ends at work, and had just thrown your daddy an early fortieth birthday party, as I thought you might arrive on his special day. There was barely anything left to do on my originally lengthy list, and all I had to do was wait, and see how and when you might reveal yourself.

I went to the *mikvah* with a few colleagues who were interested in this ritual. I felt this should be a community event, as I later learned birth often is. Before I went to undress, the other members of the group asked me my intentions, what I was going to be thinking about while immersing. I realized I had tears in my eyes when they asked me. They knew my intentions. What could I say? To be a good mother? To be worthy of the task that lay ahead? I asked them to pray for my friends, and for my sister-in-law, and anyone else they were thinking of, that God would hear their prayers and bless them with children.

I began to undress and then it hit me out of the blue. After all the prayers I had for you in the *mikvah*, and the pages and pages of words I wrote to you, I was going to immerse together with you. I had God's private audience in a double womb. And then I felt utterly calm and deeply centered. I slowly took off my jewelry, threw aside whatever I had brought, looked into the mirror, caressed you in my tummy, and smiled. The clutter and disrepair of the place seemed to disappear and I felt the holy feeling come over me once more. I felt deeply appreciative of the moment, and so thankful all at once. I showered, and still dripping let the attendant know I was ready. I revealed my large shape in all its glory, and began to descend down the seven steps as gracefully as a naked pregnant woman on the verge of childbirth might manage. The water was warm, and I allowed it to touch us everywhere. I dunked once and said the *Sh'ma*. I believe when I came up I was crying. I dunked again and said the *Shehecheyanu* (see p. 79), thanking God for your life, my life and this incredible opportunity. I dunked a third time and recited a blessing that has just been composed for using the *mikvah:*[7]

Prayer for Using the *Mikvah*

Blessed are You, Majestic Spirit of the universe, who embraces us in Your living waters.

And then I began to speak to God, my tears of gratitude mixing with the rainwater. My voice was soft and shaky, all the while it felt somehow clear and strong. I thanked God for you, and hoped that we would be good guides for your unique spirit, and good role models for you, and that you would always feel our love. I prayed that we would learn from you and grow closer together. I prayed for your life to be one of goodness, health, passion, love, family, and friendship. For you to have a good life and marriage and children of your own if that is what you wish, to have us be good and grateful parents, and to bless us with more children, siblings for you. I prayed for us to foster in you a love of Judaism. I prayed again for the timely and safe arrival of your siblings. And then I dunked once more. I prayed for an easy and spiritual healthy labor and delivery and then dunked again as if to somehow seal the deal. And then I spoke the Hebrew and English names of our friends and family who were trying to conceive.

The voices outside felt a bit more quiet now, but I knew they had been singing all along. I thanked God for them and for their prayers and wished them blessing. And then finally, I felt ready. For everything. This was to be the first of our dance in a series of movements entering into labor, the process of separating from you, and coming together in a whole new way. You were born three weeks later with shining blue eyes, and a wonderment about the world. And my journey as a mother, your mother, began.

—Amy Friedman

We encourage anyone intrigued about using the *mikvah*, but who may not be so familiar with it, to discuss it with a knowledgeable source.

Preterm Labor

When you got pregnant, you were given a due date, at which time you will be forty weeks' pregnant. At thirty-seven weeks, a pregnancy is called full-term, meaning a baby delivered after that time is unlikely to have any signs of prematurity. Approximately 10 percent of women will deliver preterm, or before thirty-seven weeks.[8] Some babies are delivered preterm because a mother goes into labor or breaks her water early; other preterm deliveries are induced for medical reasons to protect the mother or baby.

The Talmud states that a child born after six and a half months, but not before, is viable (*Yevamot* 42a). This corresponds with approximately twenty-eight weeks, which is, in fact, the point at which the fetal lungs begin to produce surfactant, a protein necessary for breathing. With the help of modern medical advances, the limit of viability has been pushed back to twenty-four weeks.

Giving birth to a premature baby is sure to be an experience full of questions and fears. The resounding call of pregnancy is the wish to have a healthy baby. A baby born preterm usually needs to spend time in the neonatal intensive care unit (NICU). We offer this reflection from Franci Levine Grater, a mother who went through this experience. At the end of the essay, Franci includes prayers she adapted for her children, which we encourage anyone in this situation to use.

Coping with Babies in the NICU

After an arduous and worrisome pregnancy that put me on bed rest at nineteen weeks and into the hospital at twenty-eight, our twins, Noah and Ella, were born at almost thirty-one weeks' gestation. We thought we were well prepared for having premature infants because I was a high-risk pregnancy since the beginning, and we had done our homework. But nothing could have prepared me for seeing my own children in the NICU environment.

The babies were small, about three pounds each, with spindly limbs and seemingly swollen torsos and heads. They each had feeding and breathing tubes down their throats; heart monitor leads stuck to the translucent skin of their chests, bellies, and legs; and lung monitors wrapped around one foot—they looked scary. Knowing how helpless they were without all the technology, and also knowing that they were experiencing discomfort and sometimes pain, made me feel helpless. The babies were constantly being tested for the various problems that can come with premature birth, and each test gave us a new reason to worry. The "one step forward, two steps back" nature of development in the NICU was particularly stressful—a baby is anemic and needs a blood transfusion, a baby isn't breathing well and needs more oxygen. Temporary setbacks in our babies' progress caused us emotional anguish over and over. The logistics of the situation were another difficulty. I was pumping milk every few hours for what became months before the babies could nurse unaided, and the daily, hour-long drive each way to the hospital was draining.

But, for me, the hardest part of Noah and Ella's time in the NICU was not being able to hold them—I couldn't hold Ella until she was three days old, and with Noah I waited a whole week. I had spent so much time when I was pregnant imagining how we would bond together, and I had read that the first moments and days are crucial to a good parent-child relationship. Having to let go of my images of nursing them to sleep in those newborn days was a huge disappointment.

My husband and I were in the NICU every day for eight weeks, and during that time all my energy and attention went to doing whatever I could to get my children healthy and home. Leaving them at the hospital night after night never got easier, and by the end I was desperate for them to be released. Ella and Noah are now vigorous sixteen-month-old toddlers, climbing on our bookcases and talking to our dog. Our weeks in the NICU are both a distant memory and ever present; I know all parents treasure their children's good health, but I am consciously grateful on a daily basis for this blessing that was once so palpably uncertain.

After Ella and Noah were born, I recited this blessing in the delivery room, adapted from the morning liturgy:

> Blessed are You, God, Spirit of the Universe, maker of light, creator of darkness, maker of peace, creator of all that is.

While I was in the hospital, I used two lines from the *Ashre* prayer as a prayer/mantra. These lines, which speak of God's abundant compassion, gave me hope during those terrible days that my two small babies would have compassion shown to them:

> Merciful and compassionate is God, patient and abounding in love, God is good to all, and compassionate toward all creation.

I said this prayer on each visit to the NICU, which has become a nightly prayer over each child:

> Shechinah, Holy Mother, bless this child [name]; protect her and shelter her beneath your wings. Help her to rest easy, help her to breathe freely, help her to grow strong. Grant her a long, healthy life of deep and abundant joy.
>
> —Franci Levine Grater

Maternal Illness in Pregnancy

Although most pregnancies are healthy, a pregnancy can in some cases bring with it health risks for the mother. This may be due to a preexisting condition, such as asthma, diabetes, or a heart condition. Other women may develop an illness particular to pregnancy, such as preeclampsia. Preeclampsia is marked by high blood pressure, swelling, and protein in the urine. Severe preeclampsia can be very dangerous for a pregnant woman. Any type of maternal illness may increase the monitoring you will need to ensure your own and the baby's safety, and force you to have an early delivery. If you are experiencing such problems, we offer this prayer:

I call to my mothers,
Sarah, Rebekah, Leah, Rachel
Wrap your strong arms around me
Give my body the support I need
So that I can reach the moment of birth
In strength, for my baby
And myself

—Sandy Falk

Almost There

We began this book by using the image of sitting in the palm of God's hand while waiting for Sandy to go into labor. If you are in the last stages of the third trimester we trust you will know what we mean. How does one wait for a radically life-changing experience? We spent some of those weeks before the delivery "nesting," that is, clearing out our guest room so that it would be empty to be used as the nursery. And making what was our office into our office/guest room. And painting, and fixing things around the house. Before this time in our lives, we fixed things in our home only when they got to the stage of absolute danger. But it felt as if we had to have everything in place for the delivery to happen.

And we saw movies. We were prescient enough to figure out that we were going to go into a movie-free zone for the next year taking care of a baby, so we saw anything that was playing. And we worried. We worried whether everything was going to be okay, and we prayed that everything was going to be okay, and we hoped that we would make good parents and that Dan would learn how to change a diaper. And we waited, sitting in God's hands, waiting to be placed into our new lives.

4

Labor and Delivery

When Sandy was a child, her older brother would sometimes trick her into going on roller coasters. He would assure her that the ride would be short with no big ups and downs. As the roller-coaster car started to roll slowly uphill, and kept going up and up and up, she would realize that she had been duped again. When she began to feel terrified about the ride ahead, Sandy's father would give her this advice: "Open your eyes and scream."

If you are pregnant and nearing delivery, you probably don't need to ask what this story has to do with you. You are about to embark on one of life's most thrilling, terrifying, and rewarding rides. When you go into labor, or arrive for a planned induction or Cesarean section, you begin this sacred journey.

We are used to navigating and controlling the world by using our minds. Laboring and delivering your baby will draw you into an undeniably physical realm. This encounter may exalt you, as you experience the surging pain of contractions, feel the blood pumping through your veins, and realize that a living child will emerge from your body; it will also utterly humble you. Weaving a spiritual thread into your labor can help you embrace and celebrate this process—the unique, profound experience that is birth.

In this chapter, we give you resources to help spiritually support you and your partner as you move through your birth process.

When Will I Go into Labor?

Fanny Neruda, a German Jewish poet in the nineteenth century, captures the expectant feelings of a mother-to-be in the following poem:[1]

Prayer on the Approach of
Accouchement [Delivery]

O my God! Soon, soon approaches the great hour
when I shall give birth to another being,
According to Thy wise ordination. O God!

Thou knowest my weakness, Thou wilt pardon me
That I look toward that hour with dread and anxiety
For Thou, Omniscient One, alone knowest
What that hour shall be unto me . . .

—Fanny Neruda

On your due date, you will be forty weeks' pregnant. Forty weeks is simply an estimate of when you may deliver. Only 4 percent of women deliver exactly on their due date.[2] This may come as a surprise, given how many people assume that their due date is absolutely written in stone. At thirty-seven weeks, a pregnancy is full-term, and delivery at any time after this is safe for your baby. Approximately 10 percent of women will deliver preterm, or before thirty-seven weeks (see the previous chapter for a discussion of preterm birth).[3] If you pass your due date, you may find that your phone starts to ring off the hook with well-meaning friends and relatives asking, "Did you deliver yet?" You may start wishing that you lived in France, where a woman's stated due date is at forty-two weeks' gestation.

When you reach thirty-seven weeks, you enter a wonderful, unpredictable phase of your life. Approaching this great unknown makes many women and their partners feel uneasy. You may be a planner, used to having much greater control over your everyday activities. Awaiting labor is the first great step in your inauguration as a parent, a path that will surprise you again and again.

What initiates labor? This is still one of the great mysteries of medicine. In other animal species, the level of the hormone progesterone drops precipitously just before labor begins. This is not true for humans. Some researchers posit that the fetus may emit a chemical messenger that triggers the entire process. We do know that, if necessary, labor can be induced using substances called prostaglandins and oxytocin, both of which are hormones that your body releases naturally during the labor process. Some women have medical reasons that make labor induction necessary.

If you are getting impatient for your labor to start, you may want to consult pregnancy books that describe using nipple stimulation and castor oil, among other suggestions.

The Rabbis describe the initiation of labor with the metaphor of a house with closed doors. "Just as there are doors to a house, so there are doors to a [pregnant] woman...just as there are keys to a house, so there are a keys to a [pregnant] woman...just as there are hinges [on the doors] of a house, so there are hinges on a [pregnant] woman [which will open up her womb]" (*Leviticus Rabbah* 14:4). The Rabbis believed that the "doors are opened" when the fetus reaches the upper chamber of the uterus. As we discussed earlier, the Talmud says that during the first trimester the fetus lives in the lowest chamber of the womb, during the second trimester it is in the middle chamber, and in the third trimester it is in the upper chamber. Labor begins when the fetus turns downward toward delivery, and this turning is the cause of a woman's labor pains (*Niddah* 31b). (The Rabbis did not have a good sense of anatomy in this regard; this is *not* the cause of labor pains.)

The Rabbis observed, as we do now, that labor and delivery occur roughly at the end of nine months. However they also saw babies born at the end of eight months who survived. To account for this difference, the Rabbis believed there were two types of "creations" (as odd as this may sound). Most fetuses are created to be born after nine months, but some are created to reach viability after seven months. It was concluded that fetuses who survived birth at eight months were actually created to mature at seven months, but stayed in the womb an extra month.[4] Our sense of the pregnancy calendar has been greatly refined since the time of the Rabbis, but it is, of course, still a mystery as to when exactly you will deliver.

As you enter the final weeks of pregnancy and you gear yourself up for labor, we offer the following prayer, to be said starting at thirty-seven weeks, which asks God to bring you to labor safely:

Prayer on the Verge of Labor

Adonai, *ruach ha'olam*
God, spirit of the world
Thank you for bringing me to this point
I am healthy, I am strong
My heart beats, my blood flows, my child moves
    inside my body
Ha-rachaman
God, full of compassion
Your ways are mysterious
Bring me through this time
And to the moment of birth
Adonai, *rachamei tiftach*
God, open my womb
Bring my child, healthy
Into the world

—Sandy Falk

The First Stage of Labor: Moving through the Red Sea

Many women ask, "How will I know when I am in labor?" Labor, like love, is unmistakable. You will already have experienced occasional contractions throughout your third trimester. Labor is defined as the combination of painful contractions and cervical dilation. For most women, contractions with the power to dilate your cervix should be so painful that you will not be able to speak while they occur and should come every five minutes for two or more hours.

Some women do rupture their amniotic membranes, or "break their water," before going into labor, so if you think this may have happened, call your midwife or obstetrician. This is what happened to Sandy. She went into labor on a Friday night. She had had Shabbat dinner at the house of the ninety-five-year-old grandmother of a friend (who still claims that her chicken should be given credit). At 1:00 A.M., she awakened suddenly, ran to the bathroom, and a flood of fluid rushed out. There must have been a pressure shift that woke her up. In fact, it is common labor and delivery lore that barometric-pressure shifts cause women to rupture their membranes. (Anecdotally, when the weather outside has that expectant feel right before a storm, it seems that many women do break their water.)

As the gush of fluid continued, we called the nurse, who told us to wait a few hours and then come in. There were no trumpets or shofars blasting, but this was it. Our world was about to be remade, and it was heralded by a small flood.

In the first stage of labor, the contractions and the pressure of the baby's head will cause your cervix to dilate. This is yet another wonder of pregnancy. The uterus consists mainly of muscle. The cervix, the lowest portion of the uterus, contains less muscle and more of a protein called collagen. Throughout your pregnancy, until labor begins, your cervix has stayed closed to keep the fetus inside. As labor approaches, the cervix ripens; its collagen breaks down and rearranges itself so that the cervix can now soften, shorten (efface), and dilate.

Many readers of the Torah have noted that the labor and delivery process seems uncannily similar to the miracle of the Red Sea, which opened to allow the Israelites to pass and then closed upon the Egyptians. Just as a fetus moves through a narrow passage to life, so the Israelites who were in *Mitzrayim*, the biblical name for Egypt but also meaning "the narrow place," left from the narrow place to new life. It may be difficult to remove Cecil B. DeMille and Charlton Heston visuals from your mind, but the Red Sea imagery is almost unmistakable as a birth canal: A path is cleared through water (amniotic fluid), and the walls of the sea (the cervix) open to allow the Israelites (the baby) to be birthed into freedom. They emerge on the other side of the path singing (screaming) with unrestrained emotion (the first moments of a baby's life). Some time later the uterine walls again open and close, forcing out the placenta (the Egyptians), at one time a crucial part of the fetus's existence, now obsolete as the baby is free to be on its own.

We encourage you to hold on to this image of God parting the waters as a focus for your birthing experience. You are the conduit for a miraculous experience. As the Israelites must have feared entering the sea but emerged triumphant, singing joyously of the great redemption, so you too will take your fears with you into this process but will, with God's help, emerge to sing joyfully of the miracle of life.

Damn Snake, Damn Eve: The Pain of Labor

Birth is transformative. A woman who has gone through pregnancy and delivery is transformed by the awesome power of having human life come through her. There may not be a more profound experience than that of one being growing inside another and then coming into the world.[5] It is an unfortunate fact, though, that during this transformative act, women suffer pain. God seems to have designed the system in a rather poor way if the goal was to maximize reproduction! Birth is difficult for the body. We hope that your experience of pregnancy is a profound one and that any pain is balanced by the joys of a healthy baby.

Biblically speaking, the pain of labor is the serpent's fault. At some point in your labor, you may find yourself cursing the snake who coaxed Eve into eating from the forbidden tree in the garden, "And to the woman He [God] said, 'I will make most severe your pangs in childbirth, in pain you shall bear children'" (Genesis 3:16). The Talmud warns against women in labor cursing their husbands about the pain they are in, declaring that they are never going to sleep with them again (*Niddah* 31b). You may find yourself cursing neither the snake, nor Eve, nor your partner, but just cursing, period.

In the Bible a few terms for labor pains are used. We find this verse in First Samuel: "*Tzirim* [labor pains] came over the birthing woman" (1 Samuel 4:19). *Tzirim* has been interpreted as "labor pains" or the "throes of labor"; elsewhere it is translated as "door hinges" (Isaiah 13:8). A woman having labor pains is also called a *cholah* in the Bible (Jeremiah 4:31). Labor is referred to as *chol*, that is, "to turn oneself in a circle." The name may come from the idea that a woman in labor walks back and forth repeatedly, as if in a circle. Another biblical term for labor pains is *chavalim*, from the root *chaval*, or "to tie together." This word probably derives from the feelings of the contractions, that is, the feeling of being in knots.[6]

Throughout the ages there have been any number of Jewish folk remedies to ease the pain of labor and induce delivery. Egyptian Jews used to write the name of the woman in labor on a coin and then put it under her tongue. In Warsaw, Jews used to put a coin on the laboring woman's belly, so the fetus would see it and hurry out. Jews from Afghanistan would collect rainwater on the seventh day of Passover for a laboring woman to drink; eastern European Jews would give a woman water from a crossroads. In the Middle Ages, Jews used to write a magic formula on the four corners of a sheet, then wash the sheet and give the wash water to the woman to drink. As a good omen to ease delivery, the knots on a woman's garments were loosened and the doors to her house were opened. In some communities, a shofar was blown on behalf of the laboring woman. Ingesting animal organs, drinking a potion of cemetery dirt, having incense burned underneath the labor bed, and wearing an amulet made of seven-year-old matzah were just a few of the ways Jews have tried to hasten delivery and alleviate the pain of childbirth.[7]

Two rather interesting customs to help a laboring woman give birth involve the use of the Torah. In some Sephardic communities, it was the custom to bring a Torah scroll right into the laboring woman's room and put it on her belly. There was some disagreement as to whether this was an appropriate act. Some Rabbis contended that it was a desecration of the Torah to use it like an amulet in the room of a birthing women. So it was permitted that only the Torah ark be opened when a woman went into labor, and prayers and psalms were recited in the synagogue for the woman's well-being.[8] Another custom in widespread use was to tie a thread from a laboring woman's hand or bed to the Torah ark as the ark is opened, so the womb will supposedly open for the fetus to come out.[9]

Although we presume you do not have easy access to a Torah or a thread long enough to reach a Torah ark, it is interesting to note that delivery was considered to be a time of such holiness and profound mystery that the Torah itself could be present for the delivery. You may wish to utilize some element of these folk customs as you prepare spiritually for your delivery.

An Etrog a Day Keeps the Pain Away: A Jewish Folk Custom for Easing the Pain of Labor

Another well-known Jewish folk custom to ease the pain of delivery was developed in eastern Europe. On the seventh day of Sukkot, called *Hoshanah Rabbah*, a pregnant women would bite the end, the *pitom*, off an *etrog* (a citrus fruit similar to a lemon). The prayer that accompanied the ritual first appeared in a book called the *Tzenerene*, a seventeenth-century book of biblical commentary written in Yiddish and specifically for women.

The source of this curious ritual goes back to the Garden of Eden. The Torah tells us that because Eve ate from the forbidden fruit, all women thereafter are cursed with pain during childbirth. Jewish commentators have long debated exactly what kind of fruit it was that Eve actually ate. Although most of us have been taught that Eve ate an apple, the Torah itself says only that Eve ate a fruit. The Rabbis offer many different fruits as the possible candidate, including an *etrog*. Because of the importance of the *etrog* during Sukkot, it might have been natural for the Rabbis to believe that this special fruit was dangling seductively from the Tree of Knowledge of Good and Evil.

In this ritual, the pregnant women takes the *etrog*, bites off the *pitom*, and spits it out to show that if she had been in the Garden she would not have eaten the fruit. Thus, the curse of a painful labor would never have come into being, and women would give birth, in the words of the *Tzenerene*, as "easy as a hen lays an egg."

Here is the prayer asking for an easy childbirth after biting off the end of an *etrog*:

Prayers for an Easy Childbirth

Lord of the world, because Eve ate of the apple, all of us women must suffer such great pangs as to die. Had I been there, I would not have had any enjoyment from [the fruit]. Just so, now I have not wanted to render the *etrog* unfit during the whole seven days when it was used for a *mitzvah*.[10] But now, on *Hoshanah Rabbah,* the *mitzvah* is no longer applicable, but I am [still] not in a hurry to eat it. And just as little enjoyment as I get from the stem of the *etrog* would I have gotten from the fruit that you forbade.[11]

Prayers and Psalms for Labor and Delivery

It is said that there are no atheists in foxholes, and this may also be the case in delivery rooms. Prayer at this moment may bring strength or inner peace or divine help.

The following prayers are a mix of contemporary prayers and traditional psalms associated with labor and delivery. You and your partner may wish to begin reciting these as your contractions begin. As labor becomes more difficult, you may ask your partner or birth coach to support you by reading them aloud. You may wish to recite only a few sentences from the prayers and repeat them over and over as a mantra. The most effective prayers are often the ones that come straight from your heart, so we also encourage you to pray spontaneously (out loud if you are able), or recite words you have written down prior to labor to pray at this moment.

- **Psalm 121:** This is referred to as "The Psalm of Ascents." It has traditionally been associated with labor and was inscribed upon plaques and displayed in delivery rooms.[12] The psalm speaks of God's protection from harm.

The Psalm of Ascents

I lift up my eyes to the mountains. What is the source of my help?
My help comes from Adonai, maker of heaven and earth.
God will not let your foot give way; your Protector will not slumber.
The Guardian of Israel neither slumbers nor sleeps.
God is your guard, God is your protection close at hand.
The sun will not strike you by day nor the moon by night.
God will guard you from all harm.
God will guard your soul, your going and your coming, now and forever.

- **Psalm 126:** There is a traditional connection between this psalm and labor, the core of which is found in the verse, "Those who sow in tears will reap in joy." This image has been taken as a reference to the pain of labor leading to the joy of birth. In general, the psalm addresses the exile of the Jewish people after the destruction of the Temple.

A Song of Ascents

When God brought back the captives of Zion, we were like dreamers.
Then was our mouth filled with laughter and our tongue with singing, then they said among the nations, "God has done great things for them."
God has done great things for us; we are glad.

Turn our captivity, O God, like the springs in the desert.
Those who sow in tears will reap in joy.
One who goes weeping on their way, bearing a bag of
   seed, shall come back with a joyful shout carrying his
   sheaves.

◆ **An eighteenth-century prayer:** This prayer is found in
the Italian prayer book for the married woman.

A Prayer for Deliverance

Open the wall of my womb so that I may bear at the proper
time this child who is within me—at a time of blessing and
salvation.

   May this child be vital and healthy.

   May I not struggle only to achieve emptiness, may I not
labor in vain, God forbid. Because You alone hold the key
to life, as it is written,

   "And God remembered Rachel and listened to her and
opened her womb" (Genesis 30:22).

   Therefore take pity on my entreaty.

   From the very depths of my heart I call to You. I raise
my voice to You, God. Answer me from the heights of
your holiness. Selah. [13]

◆ **A contemporary prayer:** This prayer comes from the
Reconstructionist Rabbinical Association Rabbi's Manual. [14]

Prayer to the Divine Midwife

May the Deliverer, who in times of trouble answers those
who call for divine help, accept my prayer as I struggle in
labor. With graciousness as deep and as wide as the sea,
God remembered my mothers and blessed them with children. So may God remember and tend to me now.
Through these labor pains my heart trembles and calls out.
My gaze is fixed upon the Eternal, my God. My hand
reaches for the divine midwife whose tender care will help
me through my sore distress. May God see my pain, and
remember my tears, and grant my petition. May my prayer
be welcome, and may I be granted relief and comfort. The

Merciful One will deliver me. The Compassionate One will return my health and vigor and well-being. The Kind One will restore my former strength. My body will be refreshed anew.

Kavvanot (Intentions) for Labor and Delivery

There is no hard and fast distinction between a prayer and a *kav-vana*, intention. In this section we are using the term *kavvana* to denote a short prayer that can be memorized. You can utilize these *kavvanot* as a point of focus as labor becomes more intense.

צֵא אַתָּה וְכָל־הָעָם אֲשֶׁר־בְּרַגְלֶיךָ וְאַחֲרֵי־כֵן
אֵצֵא.

Tze atah v'khol ha'am asher b'raglekha, v'acharei-chein eitze.

"Leave, you and all the people who follow you, and after that I will go..." (Exodus 11:8)

This verse from the Torah has been used by Jews since the Middle Ages as an incantation to ease delivery. In this verse, Moses tells Pharaoh that after the tenth plague, Pharaoh will be begging Moses and the Israelites to leave Egypt. The verse was used presumably because it speaks of "going out," even though in the biblical context it did not refer to the birth of a baby. The Exodus from Egypt is, however, a type of birth story in which the enslaved Israelites are birthed as free people.[15]

כָּל הָעוֹלָם כֻּלוֹ
גֶשֶׁר צַר מְאֹד.
וְהָעִקָּר לֹא לְפַחֵד כְּלָל.

Kol ha'olam kulo gesher tzar me'od. V'ha'ikar lo lefached klal.

The world is a very narrow bridge. The most important thing is not to be afraid.

Rebbe Nachman of Breslov was a Chasidic master who understood life as a tension between joy and pain. He counseled his disciples that joy was essential, but he also counseled them to spend some time every morning expressing their pain to God. Such a thinker's wisdom is appropriate to the labor process, which is perhaps the ultimate experience of joy and pain. This is among his most famous statements, which can be chanted as a song.

כֹּל הַנְּשָׁמָה תְּהַלֵּל יָה הַלְלוּיָה.

Kol haneshama t'halleil Yah, Halleluyah!

Let every breath praise God, Halleluyah! (Psalm 150:6)

As the last line of the last psalm in the Book of Psalms, this is often used as a *kavvana* to focus energy. It speaks of all that breathes praising God, and because at the time of labor there is such a focus on breathing, there is a natural inclination to use this psalm as a *kavvana*. This psalm may also be chanted as a song.

אֵל נָא רְפָא נָא לָה.

El na refa na la.

Please God, please heal her. (Numbers 12:13)

This is a verse from the Book of Numbers. In this prayer, Moses calls on God to heal his sister Miriam from a leprosy-like disease that has been inflicted upon her by God as a punishment. This is the first occurrence of spontaneous prayer in the Torah. Although pregnancy is clearly not a punishment, the verse is the most basic cry for help and healing in all of Jewish liturgy.

The Second Stage of Labor: Pushing and Delivery

The second stage of labor begins when a woman reaches full cervical dilation, that is, ten centimeters. Up to this point the mighty uterus did the work, and your job, or perhaps the job of your epidural anesthetic, was to bring yourself through the pain. Now you must work with your uterus to deliver your baby. Your birth support team— your partner, *doula*, nurse, midwife, doctor, or some combination of these people—will be very important to you during this phase.

Pushing can occur in any position. A woman can choose to squat, kneel on her hands and knees, lie on her side, or lie on her back.

In the Torah, there is a mention of a birthing stool called an *ovnayim*, literally "two stones." This refers to a special type of stool with a hole in the middle that a woman in labor straddles. In the famous passage where Pharaoh decrees the destruction of all Israelite baby boys, it says that Pharaoh spoke to Shifra and Puah, the midwives for the Israelites, telling them to "look on the *ovnayim*" to see whether the baby was a boy or a girl (Exodus 1:16). *Ovnayim* is an interesting word because it also refers to the stone upon which a potter throws clay. This evocative image suggests not only the position of a laboring woman but also equates giving birth with an artistic process of creation.

There are also biblical references to giving birth upon another woman's knees. In the case of Rachel, her handmaid, Bilhah, gave birth upon her knees (Genesis 30:3), using Rachel as a birth stool. We are to understand this statement both literally and figuratively. It was not uncommon throughout history, Jewish and otherwise, for women to sit on other women as birthing stools. Figuratively, this act signified that the child was symbolically born to Rachel.

Cesarean Section

Julius Caesar is reputed to be the first child born via surgery, hence the appellation. Until the modern era of anesthesia and antibiotics, Cesarean sections were performed to save a baby only when the mother had already died in childbirth. Today a C-section may be scheduled if an attempt at vaginal delivery is deemed too risky for the mother or baby or if the mother has had a previous C-section and does not wish to attempt a vaginal delivery. A C-section may also be recommended if labor does not progress or if the fetus shows distress during labor.

C-sections have been the center of various debates. Are doctors too willing to do C-sections? Alternatively, should a woman be able to choose a C-section, even without a medical reason? Should a woman who has had a C-section be able to attempt a subsequent vaginal delivery? The answers to these questions are beyond the scope of this book, but we would like to discuss the more personal side of these issues.

Some women who have a C-section feel that they have failed or have been deprived of the birth experience for which they had hoped. Recently, Sandy saw a patient who felt she had failed. She said, "Why couldn't I push my baby out in time? I feel like less of a woman." Sandy and she reviewed what had happened in detail; it seemed that the baby was in real danger and that there had been no other safe option in her case. Sandy's patient finally realized that a C-section was a life-saving operation for the baby. Like all women who need to have a C-section, she is not a failure; on the contrary, the delivery was a success because she and the baby are both healthy.

This book is written with the premise that labor and delivery can be more than just a physical experience, that through both the body and the soul you can fully experience the miracle of birth. And even if the physical details of your delivery are not what you planned for, the miracle is still the same. If you have a C-section, you are certainly not a failure, and your birth experience is not lost—it is just different. The road to parenthood is full of surprises, and what kind of birth you have is just one of the turns in the path.

If you know you will need a C-section, the following prayer may help prepare you:

Prayer Before a Cesarean Section

Let there be light
And there was light
Moments of creation
Can come suddenly,
My child
Soon, you will leave my womb
You will come into being
There will be a you and a me
As God parted the waters
We, too, will have help
I pray for the strength of our helpers
Guide me through this miraculous opening
Let us arrive, joyfully, on the other side
To the sound of timbrels

—Sandy Falk

The Moment of Delivery

Our son Naftali came into the world screaming at the top of his lungs. The pediatrician called out, "He's a wild man." Dan thought that the quiet and purring baby he expected must have been switched in *utero* with this screaming wild thing with a belly cord. We have a few pictures that Dan took of Naftali at age five seconds. In one photo, his face is contorted with screams, he is coated with newborn baby gook, and he looks a little cold. It is by far the ugliest and the most astoundingly beautiful photograph we have. Delivery is amazing, incomparable to anything else in life, perhaps beyond words. The moment of delivery is, to use Rabbi Abraham Joshua Heschel's oft-quoted phrase, one of radical amazement.

Jewish tradition suggests only two brief blessings at the moment of delivery, perhaps because the moment is so overwhelming that one does not need a lot of outside words or formal rituals to be made intensely aware of God's presence. There is a tradition of saying a short blessing at the moment of delivery, a thank-you to God for having survived this most difficult time with mother and baby alive.

בָּרוּךְ אַתָּה יְיָ אֱלֹהֵינוּ מֶלֶךְ הָעוֹלָם, הַטוֹב וְהַמֵּטִיב.

Barukh atah Adonai, eloheinu melekh ha'olam, hatov v'hameitiv.

Blessed are You, Adonai our God, ruler of the universe, who is good and does good.

בָּרוּךְ אַתָּה יְיָ אֱלֹהֵינוּ מֶלֶךְ הָעוֹלָם, שֶׁהֶחֱיָנוּ וְקִיְּמָנוּ וְהִגִּיעָנוּ לַזְּמַן הַזֶּה.

Barukh atah Adonai, eloheinu melekh ha'olam, shehecheyanu, v'kiyimanu, v'higiyanu, lazman hazeh.

Blessed are You, Adonai our God, ruler of the universe, Who gives us life, sustains us, and enables us to reach this moment.

(Traditionally, the *Hatov v'hameitiv* blessing is used for a boy and the *Shehecheyanu* blessing for a girl, but in our view the blessings can be used regardless of gender, if desired.)

Another possible blessing to be said at this moment is found in the Reconstructionist Rabbinical Association Rabbi's Manual. This blessing is gender-neutral in its reference to God.

נְבָרֵךְ אֶת עֵין הַחַיִּים עוֹשֶׂה מַעֲשֶׂה בְּרֵאשִׁית.

Nevarekh et Ein Hachayim oseh ma'aseh v'reishit.

Let us bless the Source of Life, who performs the mysteries of creation.

The Third Stage of Labor: Delivering the Placenta

The final stage of labor is the delivery of the placenta, or the afterbirth. The placenta forms when the developing embryo burrows into the wall of the uterus, and it provides the conduit for exchange of oxygen and nutrients between the mother and the fetus through the umbilical cord. An incredible array of hormones that support the pregnancy are also produced by the placenta.

The Talmud says that after delivery, the placenta should be pre-served in a bowl with oil, straw, or sand, depending on the wealth of its bearer (*Niddah* 27a). This custom reflects a belief in the symbiot-ic connection between the placenta and the child. By preserving the placenta in this way, parents were keeping it warm in the hope that it would have some magical effect on the child.

The Palestinian Talmud goes further and says that after a few days the preserved placenta should be buried in the earth and the parents should take an oath (*Shabbat* 18:16), pledging to the earth that the body of the new person will be returned when he/she dies. One scholar who has researched this custom comments, "This . . . statement expresses a very old and important folk idea: on the very day of one's birth, a person must give a pledge to the earth to assure her that he will return to her when he dies. A person is born of earth and to the earth they return. So that the earth will wait patiently . . . the afterbirth is buried as a pledge."[16] Some modern Jewish women have chosen to renew this ancient custom of burying the placenta with that same intention of returning to the earth that which belongs to the earth.

Birth Pangs of the Messiah

As a final note on labor and delivery, we have a few words about theology, the existence of evil, and the redemption of the world. There is a rabbinic concept called "the birth pangs of the Messiah" that has been used to explain why the Jewish people have suffered so much pain throughout history. The Rabbis use the metaphor of a woman in labor to say that nothing can be born without a type of death. For something to be born, something else has to die. A seed may eventually grow into an apple tree, but for the apple tree to grow, the seed needs to cease being a seed; it must die in a certain way for the tree to be born. Before a woman gives birth, she must suffer a type of death from the great pains she is enduring. A midrash says, "While squatting upon the birth stool, ninety-nine of her groans despair unto death, while only one calls out for life" (Tanchuma, *Tazria* 6).

The Rabbis use this metaphor to say that the pain of the Jewish people is like a labor pain; it is just a prelude to a birth. In the case of the Jewish people, the pains are leading to the birth of the Messiah. The ramifications of such a theology are quite provocative. This idea suggests that the great sufferings of the Jewish people have meaning. Jewish suffering is necessary for the redemption of the world to occur.

We do not suggest that you think about the pain of the Jewish people while you are trying to give birth; your own pain is quite enough. Rather, we seek to sustain you with another understanding of how the pains of labor are necessary for the birth to happen. God is acting through this pain to create new life. And as you are grabbing for ice chips, or an epidural, or both, know that after ninety-nine painful groans, the last one will be, with God's help, for life.

5

The Days after Birth

Mazel tov! You are now a parent! From the moment that your loved ones first wished you *b'sha-ah tovah*, you have made perhaps the longest, the most joyful, and the most arduous journey of your life. We hope that you have arrived healthy and are holding a healthy baby in your arms. If, unfortunately, you are still facing special concerns for yourself or your child, we hope for you a *refuah shleimah*, a speedy and healthy recovery.

The first days of parenthood are filled with wonder. Counting fingers, toes, days of life, diaper changes; this is a time of life when it is easy to feel that you are in the presence of miracles. We encourage you to make an effort to experience each magical moment fully.

This time also has its challenges. Remember that your body has just gone through a major physical experience. In many cultures, to help the healing process, a new mother goes through a period of separation or has specific restrictions on what she is allowed to do or to eat. The Rabbis of the Talmud believed that the recovery of a postpartum woman was of such importance that the laws of Shabbat could be broken to gather wood for her, if she wishes a fire to keep her warm (*Shabbat* 129a). Give yourself time to recover. If you have a community of friends and family or a synagogue, consider asking for help with meals, but also remember to set limits on visitors so that you can rest. Above all, be choosy about taking advice but open to accepting help.

Bringing Your Baby Home

Remember that old custom of a groom carrying his bride across the threshold of their home the first time they enter it after their marriage? There is something about coming home as a new family for the first time that naturally calls out for a ritual or a prayer. When you bring home a baby from the hospital, there is a profound understanding that this is a special moment. Maybe it is just a feeling of thanks for having brought a child home. Maybe it is the feeling that "home" has just been transformed in an unimaginable way. Many families have personal stories about being greeted by ribbons and pictures and signs saying, "Welcome Home!"

The following is a prayer for this moment of return. If you have a *mezuzah* hanging, we suggest gathering together under the *mezuzah*, spending one moment in quiet accepting this miracle and reciting the prayer.

Prayer for Bringing a Baby Home
for the First Time

As this child has been nurtured in the womb, so may we continue to feel Your caring presence in our home. As we attend to his/her needs, grant us protection and guidance.

May this home be a shelter for our child, a place where arms shall cradle him/her and voices sing lullabies, where hands will uphold him/her and eyes delight in watching him/her grow.

In this home may we reach out to each other in love.

May our hearts be turned to each other.

May we create bonds of trust and care that will keep us close as we grow together as a family.

Bless us, Nurturing One, all of us together in your light. For in Your light, Embracing One, You have given us the Torah of life, loving-kindness, justice, blessing, caring, life, and *shalom*.[1]

Welcoming a Jewish Baby

From a Jewish point of view, the highlight of the days after birth is, for a boy, the *b'rit milah*, the circumcision ceremony that occurs on the eighth day after birth, or for a girl, the *b'rit bat*, the covenant ceremony that can occur on a day of one's choosing. This ceremony marks the official inclusion of the baby into the Jewish community. Traditionally, one does not even announce the new baby's name until the *b'rit*. We will not go into detail here about planning the *b'rit milah* or the *b'rit bat*, but we recommend that you read *The New Jewish Baby Book: Names, Ceremonies & Customs—A Guide for Today's Families* (Jewish Lights) by Anita Diamant, which has become the standard book on the subject for non-Orthodox Jews, and *Celebrating Your New Jewish Daughter: Creating Jewish Ways to Welcome Baby Girls into the Covenant* (Jewish Lights) by Debra Nussbaum Cohen.

There is a custom among observant Jews called *shalom zakhar* (greeting the male child), which recognizes the new baby before the eighth day. On the Friday night before the *b'rit milah*, a party is held, usually at the home of the new parents, to welcome the child into the world. Fruits and cake are served to wish a sweet life for the child. You may consider extending this tradition to honor the arrival of a baby girl.[2]

Older Siblings Welcoming a New Baby

With the excitement and attention focused on the new baby, older siblings often feel left out of the process, and they may start acting out at this time. Child experts say to watch for older children to regress at this time in an attempt to vie for attention with the newborn. Older siblings should be given the opportunity to share in the blessings of the new baby; even if they are worried about sharing their parents with someone else, they will have feelings of excitement about the new person in their lives. The following essay by Rabbi Michelle Robinson addresses this issue and gives suggestions for blessings an older child might say upon welcoming a new baby into the house.

It Better Be a Sister

I remember waking up one morning in our home in New Jersey to find an elderly woman sitting in our living room. "Where are mom and dad?" I asked. "At the hospital," she answered gently. "Soon you'll hear about your new baby brother or sister." "It better be a sister," I said, "or else I'm not letting them come home."

Luckily for my parents it was a girl. I was six then, and I had very strong ideas about what this new baby would mean for my life. I remember seeing my new little sister through the glass at the nursery later that afternoon, and when she was brought home, my parents showed me they understood that she was special not just to them, but to me as well. As soon as they arrived, they seated me in a chair and let me be the first to hold her. It was a very special moment for me. I felt important, grown up. I had all sorts of things I wanted to say to this new little sister of mine. It was a moment for a blessing. But what blessing?

Our Rabbis taught that each one of us should say one hundred blessings a day. There are blessings for eating, for study, for new things. But what is the blessing for an older sibling welcoming a new baby? I'd like to suggest several possibilities.

First of all, depending on the age of the older sibling, a *Shehecheyanu* could be very appropriate. It is a blessing for new things and new experiences, and the moment when an older sibling first meets his or her brother or sister is definitely a moment filled with "newness."

There is also a beautiful blessing in our traditional compendium of blessings that the Rabbis instruct us to say upon seeing particularly beautiful people. A newborn, being one of the most beautiful of God's creations, certainly is worthy of this blessing: *Barukh atah Adonai, eloheinu melekh ha'olam, sh'Kacha lo b'olamo*. "Blessed are You, Lord our God, ruler of the universe, who has such things in your world."

Or perhaps the blessing for hearing good news fits best: *Barukh atah Adonai, eloheinu melekh ha'olam, ha'tov v'hameitiv.* "Blessed are You, Lord our God, ruler of the universe, who is good and brings good."

But what if the older sibling is not yet old enough for such detailed Hebrew blessings? The first words traditionally said by the community as we welcome a new baby at a bris are "*Barukh Ha'ba,*" meaning "Welcome." These words, while uncomplicated, are a very powerful way for a child to welcome his or her new sibling. They could be recited either at the hospital or as a way for the older sibling to welcome the new baby for the first time to the family home. This would work particularly well if the older sibling stood at or near the doorway when the new baby was brought home for the first time. Before the parents enter with the baby, they wait for the older sibling to say, "*Barukh Ha'ba*" for a boy or "*Brucha HaBa'ah*" for a girl. This gives the older sibling a sense of inclusion and importance at a time when he or she might be struggling with complicated feelings about the arrival of a newborn. These words can also be recited by a sibling at the naming or *b'rit milah* of the new baby. Of course, free-form blessings or words of welcome in English from an older sibling are always lovely to include in any naming ceremony if the older child wishes to participate in that way.

An older sibling who is too young to speak can still be included in welcoming the new baby by being asked to give the new baby a kiss or a hug at a special moment when family is gathered.

No matter what you decide is the best way for your children to participate in welcoming and blessing a new brother or sister, including them in some way will help them feel that this is a sacred moment, not only for the adults but for them as well.

—Rabbi Michelle Robinson

The Partner

Although families are different in how child care is divided, with some families hewing to a more traditional arrangement of the mother doing the bulk of the child care while the father continues to work, in our house we try to have a fully egalitarian approach to childrearing. This means Dan did not sleep either. As the partner of a birth parent, you may end up taking care of two people at once, the mother and the baby. And if you are a male birth partner, you may encounter some outside resistance to the concept that you are even capable of caring for the child.

On the second night of our son's life, a nurse came into our hospital room and saw that Sandy looked incredibly tired. The nurse announced that she was taking the baby to the nursery for the night. We protested, telling her that we would take care of our son (Dan was spending the night in the room). The nurse looked right at Dan and said, "But Sandy had a C-section and cannot get out of bed. Who is going to take care of the baby?" We let her know that Dan had been doing everything so far and that we would be just fine.

There is a biblical precedent for a man being responsible for childrearing. In the Book of Esther, the Bible tells us that Esther (Hadassah) was an orphan and her uncle Mordecai took her in as his own daughter. The Bible says that "Mordecai reared (*omen*) Hadassah, that is, Esther, since she had no mother or father" (Esther 2:7). The word *omen* is used in other places to mean "to nourish" someone; it can even mean "breast-feed." It seems implausible that the Bible is suggesting that Mordecai somehow breast-fed Esther, but the word has great implications. It connotes that Mordecai behaved as any loving mother would to a child, acting in a nourishing and supportive way. We hope that you, the partner of the birth mother, have the opportunity to act as Mordecai did, and thus share in the deep blessings of parenthood.

Prayer for Sleep

After even one day of parenthood, you may read the subheading "Prayer for Sleep" and presume we are offering a prayer for how you could get more sleep. But this prayer is to be said for your little one when he/she goes to bed.

As a new parent, one of the most anxiety-provoking occasions is when your new baby goes off to sleep. New parents spend much of their time trying to coax their babies to fall asleep, only to worry about their babies when they actually do. Sleeping newborns make all sorts of strange noises that strike fear in the hearts of their parents. You may worry that your child may be vulnerable to Sudden Infant Death Syndrome, and may run to his/her side every time he/she breathes loudly. These worries are all part of the parenting experience.

The following prayer is modeled on the traditional prayer for sleep that individuals say before going to bed. This prayer asks God to spread a "*sukkah* of peace" over the newborn, a shelter of protection to guard him/her from any harm.

Prayer for Safe Sleep

Blessed are You, God, ruler of the universe, who brings sleep to her eyes and slumber to her eyelids. God and God of my ancestors, may she lie down peacefully and wake up peacefully. Do not let her sleep be disturbed by troubling thoughts or bad dreams, and may her bed be perfect before You. Illuminate her eyes so she will not die in sleep. Blessed are You, God, who illuminates the whole world with your glory. Our God, help her to lay down in peace and awaken her to life. Spread over her your *sukkah* of peace and guide her with your good advice. Save her for the sake of your name and defend her from enemies, disease, swords, famine, and sorrow. Remove evil from in front of her and from behind her. Shelter her in the shadow of your wings, as You guard and redeem us—You are a compassionate and gracious God. Safeguard our coming and going for life and for peace now and forever. In your hand is the life of every living creature, the breath of all human flesh. In your hand we entrust her spirit, [because] You have redeemed us, God of truth.

—Aurora Mendelsohn

Lilith

Just as there are Jewish folk customs for preventing miscarriage and easing the pain of delivery, so there are customs to protect a newborn. Historically, the primary focus of these customs is Lilith. In recent years, Lilith has been embraced by Jews and non-Jews as a feminist symbol; she is certainly the only character in rabbinic literature who has ever had a women's rock festival named after her (see Sarah McLachlan's Lilith Fair, www.lilithfair.com).

Although the roots of Lilith go back to ancient Mesopotamian culture, the first extensive stories about Lilith are found in an eleventh-century book called *The Alphabet of Ben Sira,* where the author says that Adam's first wife was not Eve, but Lilith. This comes about because of a textual contradiction in the Torah. It says in Genesis 1:27: "He [God] created him, male and female, He created them." Only in the second chapter of Genesis do we meet Adam and his wife, Eve, taken from Adam's rib. The two creation stories are normally harmonized to say that the first mention in Genesis 1 tells the general story and the second mention in Genesis 2 fills in the specifics, but some commentators have seen other possibilities.

The Alphabet of Ben Sira says that the first creation refers to the creation of Adam and Lilith. In this story, Adam tries to assert his dominance over her, and she reasons that since they were created together she is his equal:

> Adam and Lilith never found peace together; for when he wished to lie with her, she took offense at the recumbent posture he demanded. "Why must I lie beneath you?" she asked.

"I was also made from dust, and am therefore your equal."
Because Adam tried to compel her obedience by force, Lilith,
in a rage, uttered the magic name of God and rose up in the
air and left him.[3]

The story continues that Lilith goes to live by the Red Sea and
refuses Adam's requests for reconciliation. Three angels visit her
and order her to go back upon pain of death. But she refuses, saying that God has given her domain over all babies from the moment
they are born until a boy turns eight days and a girl turns twenty
days: "Nonetheless, if ever I see your three names or likenesses displayed in an amulet above a newborn child, I promise to spare it."

Because of this story, Lilith is known in Jewish tradition as a
demon who steals babies and devours them, but we also learn that
an amulet has the power to drive her away. So it became a medieval
Jewish custom to hang amulets against Lilith above the bed and
over the doorposts from the time of delivery until the circumcision
(for a boy) or for twenty days (for a girl). The amulets have inscrip-
tions on them depicting or naming the three angels, Sansoi,
Sansanoi, and Samengalof, and ask for their help in protecting the
newborn.

Jewish feminists who have reclaimed Lilith celebrate Lilith's
demands for equality, and they revile the part of the story where
she is seen as a demon kidnapper of newborns. Being staunch feminists ourselves, we too reject Lilith's role as a demon, and we suggest
one way of reclaiming her for the birthing process. In these stories,
Lilith represents strength and self-sufficiency (choosing a life alone
as opposed to going back to Adam), as well as a connection with
nature (she, like Adam, is created from dust). As you recover from
your delivery, allow yourself to meditate on these aspects of Lilith.
Focus on your mental and physical strength, and see your body as a
vehicle for the awe-inspiring power of nature. In the birthing
process Lilith is a symbol of strength and nature, brought together to
raise new life.

Breast-feeding

Breast-feeding has many health advantages for both you and your baby. We encourage you to speak with your doctor or midwife about the most current research on the topic. Besides the nutritional benefits to your child, nursing can also be an incredible bonding experience, and it extends the satisfaction of giving physical support to your child that you felt during pregnancy.

If you are having trouble getting started, you are not alone. Go easy on yourself; just because something is natural does not necessarily mean it is easy. Taking a class on breast-feeding before and after you deliver is valuable. There are many books, support groups, and lactation consultants who can offer help. A good place to start is calling your local chapter of La Leche League, an international organization providing breast-feeding support .

Sandy's patients often ask her, "Does my partner need to come to the breast-feeding class?" The answer is a resounding yes. And this is not just to make your partner feel included; a knowledgeable, supportive partner is a great help in the nursing process. Your partner can help you with positioning the baby and make sure you are comfortable and are being hydrated.

We would like to pass along one small tidbit of advice to help prevent a hospital pitfall that Sandy has seen all too frequently with her patients. Lactation consultants universally recommend starting to nurse immediately after birth and to defer any contact with a bottle until breast-feeding is well established. If you are in the hospital, on your first night after delivery a well-meaning staff member may offer to give the baby a bottle so that you can get some sleep. Because bottle-feeding is much easier for babies, in the morning and the days that follow, you may find that your baby refuses to nurse. Either try to keep the baby with you during the night, or ask for the baby to be brought to you to nurse, even if that entails waking you up.

Some women will not be able to breast-feed. If this includes you, do not feel guilty: You are now a Jewish mother, and there will be plenty of other things to feel guilty about. Feeding a baby in any way is a nurturing and connective experience.

If you are able to breast-feed, you may experience emotions that you might not expect from this simple act. This is what happened to Aurora Mendelsohn, whose experience of nursing caused a profound transformation in her spiritual life. She wrote the following essay describing this transformation.[4]

God as a Breast-feeder and Other Jewish Views of Nursing

Even before I became the steward of another person's body, I was committed to the many advantages of breast-feeding over bottle-feeding. According to the American Academy of Pediatrics, nursing offers protection from many diseases and disorders, not only during the time that the mother and child actually engage in it, but throughout the remainder of *both* parties' lives. I also saw how a mother's emotional connection to her baby evolves naturally from the biological act of nursing—from the calming hormones released in both mother and baby, and from the fact that a mother cannot go more than several hours without feeding (or pumping milk for) her child, and thus cannot be separated from him or her for more than a day.

Beyond the physical and emotional benefits of breast-feeding, there was another aspect of breast-feeding which overwhelmed me and which I was not expecting. Many new parents say that while witnessing the birth of their children they feel closer to God than they have ever felt in their lives. For me it was not only the birth, but it was in nursing my child that I felt a profound connection to the sacred.

Because of this connection, I decided to do some research into what Judaism has to say about nursing, and I was delighted to discover how many positive and moving references to nursing exist in Jewish texts. Until fairly recently, nursing was, of course, a life-or-death issue: If one couldn't nurse, one's baby simply starved, unless, that is, one could afford a wet nurse. Breasts, therefore, are portrayed in the Torah, Midrash, and Talmud as a gift from God, a miracle and a blessing, whose explicit purpose is clearly to sustain life and provide nourishment.

The Rabbis of the Talmud portray the biblical Hannah, barren, offering God the following challenge:

> "Ruler of the World, among the things that You created in women, You have not made one without a purpose: eyes to see, ears to hear, a nose to smell, a mouth to speak, hands to do work, legs to walk with. These breasts that You put on my heart, God, are they not for nursing? Give me a son, then, so that I can use them!" (*Berakhot* 31b)

The Rabbis also show Abraham extolling the miracle of breast-feeding and its connection to the Divine in a midrash where he tells Sarah, "In order to hallow God's name, uncover your breast, so that all may be aware of the miracles that the Holy One has begun to perform" (*Genesis Rabbah* 53:9).

In biblical references to nursing, the act is understood as a continuation of the birthing process. After Isaac is born to a geriatric Sarah, for example, she expresses her astonishment: "Who would have said to Abraham that Sarah would nurse children? Yet I have borne Abraham a son in his old age!" (Genesis 21:7). And after we hear of the birth of Moses, the Book of Exodus loses very little time in describing Pharaoh's daughter arranging for a wet nurse, who—due to Miriam's extraordinary *chutzpah*—turns out to be the child's own biological mother (Exodus 2:7–9). Yet another validation of the role of breast-feeding comes from the prophet Hosea, who, in a fever of rhetoric, invokes upon wayward humanity one of the worst curses he can imagine: "Give them wombs that miscarry," he cries to God, "and breasts that are dry!" (Hosea 9:14).

The most powerful image of nursing in Jewish tradition is one which surprised me, but since I learned of it, has been at the center of my newfound connection with Judaism. The image is simple: God as a breast-feeder. As a nursing mother, the Book of Isaiah chapter 66:10–13, for example, thrilled me with its imagery of both Jerusalem and God as breast-feeding mothers and of burgeoning nations as ever-abundant breast milk:

Be joyful with Jerusalem, all you who love her, all you who mourn over her, that you may nurse and be satisfied with her comforting breasts, that you may suck deeply and be delighted with her bountiful breast! For this is what the Lord says: "Behold, I extend peace to her like a river; and the glory of nations like an overflowing stream. You will be suckled and carried on the hip and fondled on the knees. As a mother comforts her child, so will I comfort you."

—(66:10–13)

In the Book of Deuteronomy, there is a poetic description of God feeding God's people honey from the rock as they marched through the wilderness (Deuteronomy 32:13). The word the Torah uses though for "fed" is *vayenikehu*—to breast-feed. God made the people suckle honey from a rock. The image is evocative, poetic, and mystical. The image is also certainly more evidence that one of the metaphors the Bible has for God is The One Who Breast-feeds.

The image of God as a nursing mother provides women who breast-feed with an image of ourselves as God, and an understanding of our baby's utter dependence upon us as the extrapolated condition of all humankind. And when we as parents relieve our newborns from their helplessness and their inability to exert control over their circumstances, we identify with our babies' worldview. Indeed, hunger, cold, discomfort, and the threat of endless loneliness present themselves... at least until the All-Powerful One appears and instantly provides food and shelter, warmth and love, and a seeming ability to mind-read one's most profound needs and wishes.

When my husband is unable to console our daughter, he passes her to me, jokingly calling me "God." And, indeed, breast-feeding has presented me with a powerful new theology. It is both exhilarating and terrifying to realize a human being's complete dependence on you. My responsibilities have given me a taste of the sacred, of God's role in relation to comforting humanity, of what it means to be the one in charge—the grownup, the parent, the elder.

This image is relevant and evocative in a way that God the King is not. Through my own breasts I made a profound Jewish connection to God the Nursing Mother, to the God who extends peace to us like a river of milk, who assures us of overflowing streams when our lives depend on it, who carries us on Her hip and keeps us alive with Her nurturant breast. As I try to do for my child.

—Aurora Mendelsohn

Postpartum Depression

The postpartum period has many physical and emotional changes, and up to 70 percent of women experience the "postpartum blues."[5] Symptoms include tearfulness, anxiety, and irritation, and they usually subside within one to two weeks. It is common to have ambivalent feelings about your baby. A small percentage of postpartum women, however, experience severe depression or anxiety, even psychosis. If your feelings of depression or anxiety persist, if they interfere with your ability to function, or if you fear that you may harm yourself or your child, we urge you to contact your midwife or physician for help immediately.

Postpartum depression has been around for as long as birth itself; the Talmud, in fact, even includes a story of infanticide by a woman whom the Rabbis declare insane (*Yevamot* 47b). In periods of depression, you may wish to call upon God to rescue you from despair. At such difficult moments, Jews have traditionally turned to the Psalms for solace.

The following is Psalm 27, traditionally recited every morning in the month preceding Rosh Hashanah. The psalm alternates between feelings of strength and fear, ultimately crying out to God for help.

Psalm 27

The Lord is my light and my salvation. Whom shall I fear? The Lord is the strength of my life. Of whom shall I be afraid?

When the wicked, my enemies and my adversaries, came
   upon me to eat up my flesh, they stumbled and fell.
Though a host should encamp against me, my heart shall not
   fear; though war should rise against me, even then I will be
   confident.
One thing have I desired of the Lord, that I will seek after; that
   I may dwell in the house of the Lord all the days of my life, to
   behold the beauty of the Lord, and to frequent the Lord's
   temple.
For in the time of trouble God shall hide me in God's pavilion;
   under the cover of God's tent shall God hide me; God shall
   set me up upon a rock.
And now shall my head be lifted up above my enemies around
   me; therefore I will offer in God's tent sacrifices of joy; I will
   sing, I will make music to the Lord.
Hear, O Lord, when I cry with my voice; be gracious to me,
   and answer me.
Of You my heart said, Seek my face; your face, O Lord, will I
   seek!
Hide not your face from me; put not your servant away in
   anger; you have been my help; do not abandon me, nor for-
   sake me, O God of my salvation.
For my father and my mother have forsaken me, but the Lord
   will take me up.
Teach me your way, O Lord, and lead me on a level path,
   because of my enemies.
Do not give me up to the will of my enemies; for false witnesses
   have risen up against me, and they breathe out violence.
Were it not that I believe, I should see the goodness of the
   Lord in the land of the living.
Wait on the Lord; be of good courage, and God shall strength-
   en your heart; and wait on the Lord.

Rituals of Closure

Jewish rituals mark transitions in our lives. Weddings are the transition from being single to being married, bar/bat mitzvahs mark the
transition between childhood and the first stirrings of adulthood.

Jewish rituals accomplish this transition by hearkening back to our past lives and awakening us to a new future. The following two rituals mark the transition between pregnancy and motherhood. The recitation of *Birkat Hagomel* (the thanksgiving blessing) puts a closure on the experience of labor and delivery by thanking God for having allowed us to come through it safely. And a visit to the *mikvah*, whose waters are symbolic of new beginnings, awakens us fully to the new role of mother.

Visiting the mikvah

As we discussed on page 55, it is a custom to visit the *mikvah* after you have delivered. Traditionally, a woman goes seven days after the birth of a male child and fourteen days after the birth of a female child. We suggest waiting at least fourteen days before going to the *mikvah* — whenever you feel ready to transition into your new life as a mother and have recovered from the delivery. Some women seem to pop out of the delivery room and look as if they were ready for an evening of dancing; for others, the recovery can take months. Especially if you have had a C-section or had some significant tearing, be gentle with yourself. Remember if you have had a C-section that this is surgery, and you should not expect yourself to be jumping rope in the first few weeks. If you have delivered vaginally, you should also be gentle at first; delivering a baby is a trying experience on your body.

Going to the *mikvah* after you have fully recovered physically and spiritually from the delivery may be a wonderful way for you to embrace this next phase of your life as a mother to a newborn.

Birkat Hagomel: *thanksgiving blessing*

Birkat Hagomel is a traditional prayer of thanksgiving to be said by someone who has survived a dangerous situation, such as a journey, an illness, or a birth. Its recitation has become increasingly common in nonorthodox Jewish circles, perhaps because it responds very directly to a need of mothers to publicly give thanks for having survived childbirth physically and spiritually. *Birkat Hagomel* can be said at synagogue during the Torah service, at the *b'rit milah* or *b'rit bat*, or at a gathering specifically for the purpose of reciting this blessing.

[The new mother recites:]

בָּרוּךְ אַתָּה יְיָ אֱלֹהֵינוּ מֶלֶךְ הָעוֹלָם, הַגּוֹמֵל
לְחַיָּבִים טוֹבוֹת, שֶׁגְּמָלַנִי כָּל טוֹב.

Barukh atah Adonai, eloheinu melekh ha'olam, hagomel lechayavim tovot, shegemalani kol tov.

Blessed are You, Adonai our God, ruler of the world, who bestows kindness on the undeserving, and has bestowed on me all that is good.

(Alternative free translation: Thank you, God, for restoring my life to me.)

[Everyone present recites:]

מִי שֶׁגְּמָלֵךְ כָּל טוֹב, הוּא יִגְמְלֵךְ כָּל טוֹב. סֶלָה.
אָמֵן.

Mi shegemalekh kol tov, he yigmalekh kol tov. Selah. Amen.

May the one who bestowed favor on you continue to grant you all that is good. Selah. Amen.

The following essay by Rabbi Amy Bardack describes very powerfully her experience of reciting *Birkat Hagomel* after an arduous and dangerous delivery.

A Life-Threatening Childbirth

I did not have the birth I had expected. After thirty-six healthy weeks, I developed a severe form of preeclampsia with HELLP syndrome, a condition of high blood pressure, low blood platelets, and liver and kidney damage. I came to the doctor with a terrible backache (which was later believed to be caused by an inflamed liver) and within hours was in critical condition. The baby was removed by C-section, and for the day that followed the birth my condition remained life-threatening. Thankfully, I recovered quickly and my baby was fine. In the days after the birth, I became overwhelmed by the incomprehensible fact that I had nearly lost my life. Gratitude for my recovery was mixed with terror of what could have happened. The *b'rit milah*, circumcision, for our son was fast approaching. I was eager to celebrate the arrival of our first child and welcome him into the covenant. At the same time, I knew that the ceremony would feel false and incomplete if, amidst the joy, there were not also an acknowledgment of my close call with death.

The most fitting blessing to recite was *Birkat Hagomel*, the traditional blessing that thanks God for having survived a life-threatening situation. According to the Talmud, *Birkat Hagomel* is to be recited by four categories of people: those who have traveled by sea; those who have traveled through the desert; those who have recovered from a serious illness; and those who have been released from prison (*Berakhot* 54a). In talmudic times, these were all life-threatening experiences, so later Jewish sources generalized to say that anyone who had been through a life-threatening experience should recite this blessing.[6] In recognition of the potential danger of the birthing process, it has become common in some Jewish communities for women to recite *Birkat Hagomel* after childbirth.

Birkat Hagomel is often recited at synagogue during the Torah service, where the person who has been through the experience is called up to the Torah and recites this blessing over it. But the blessing need not be recited only in synagogue; the traditional requirement is only that one needs a *minyan* (at least ten people) to say it, although some Jewish legal experts argue that you may say it in front of even one person.[7] The requirement that other people hear the blessing means that reciting *Birkat*

Hagomel is an interesting mixture of the public and private. The recitation of the blessing in front of a group effectively announces that you have recovered from serious danger, but the exact circumstances of the danger are not expressed, thereby maintaining a measure of discretion within an otherwise public ritual.

As a rabbi, I had presided over others' recitations of *Birkat Hagomel:* people who had walked away from a serious car accident, recovered from heart surgery, or missed their flight on a plane that later crashed. I had never recited it myself. Saying it at my son's *b'rit milah,* accompanied by words of blessing and comfort from a rabbi who had been with me in the hospital, gave me fresh insight into the power of this prayer.

Birkat Hagomel gave me words to express my gratitude and my fear without dominating the celebration of my son's life. Acknowledging the danger publicly helped assimilate the reality of what I went through, breaking through the emotional numbness that often accompanies a crisis. Confronting the possibility of one's mortality can be powerfully isolating. The communal response to *Birkat Hagomel* and the requirement that it be said in front of others affirmed my connection to community precisely at a time when I might have felt most existentially alone. Hearing my friends and family (and even my obstetrician, who was in attendance) bless me in return reminded me of the support I had in the healing process.

I realized that reciting *Birkat Hagomel* did not benefit me alone. Introducing the blessing, my rabbi friend spoke personally about her own gratitude for my recovery. The communal response within *Birkat Hagomel* enabled my friends and loved ones to voice their relief that I had survived. Having a ritual that acknowledged the traumatic nature of the birth allowed all who were present to welcome my son into the covenant more fully and joyously.

—Rabbi Amy Bardack

6

From This Narrow Place, I Call to You:
Pregnancy Loss

We wish that no one needed to turn to this page. If you have found your way to this difficult place, we recognize your grief. Experiencing a loss can feel lonely, but you are not alone in having experienced such sadness. Unfortunately, 30 percent of pregnancies end in loss.[1] A pregnancy loss is a difficult experience, and it may make you feel as if you were being abandoned or punished by God, how else to explain that such a wonderful and precious thing was taken away from you seemingly for no reason? You may feel angry and you will certainly feel sad. The loss of a pregnancy at any point is a loss of an expected life, a potential member of your family.

Pregnancy loss is surprisingly common in the first trimester. Depending on how early a pregnancy is confirmed, approximately 20 percent of pregnancies miscarry before fourteen weeks. If you ask every woman you know, you will find that many have had a miscarriage. Unfortunately, many people do not talk about miscarriage, forming a sorority of silence. It is common practice to wait to go public with news about a pregnancy until twelve to fourteen weeks. While this makes it possible to protect your privacy in case of a miscarriage, it also sometimes makes it difficult for you to reach out for support to friends and family.

Pregnancy loss in the second trimester is tragic and often occurs without warning. By this point, you had probably put aside your first-trimester worries about miscarriage. You had given yourself permission to make plans, to announce the news. A second trimester loss can be a cruelly sad experience. The second trimester is also referred to as the mid-trimester, and this sense of being in the middle complicates the experience of pregnancy loss at this time. You are early enough in a pregnancy that friends and family may not fully understand that this is not a typical miscarriage, yet you are far enough along that the physical experience of loss may include a more complicated procedure or an actual labor and delivery.

Pregnancy is a vulnerable time, and loss of the fetus can occur until the end, or even shortly after birth. When a pregnancy passes twenty weeks, you have already felt your baby move, and you have made an intimate connection with your future child. Sometimes a fetus will die suddenly in utero, or during labor; other babies die shortly after birth due to prematurity or other complications. There are no words to describe such a loss. Your mourning will be profound. Friends and family may not know what to say to you or how to comfort you.

It is important to know that miscarriage and stillbirth are not your fault. You will almost certainly start searching your memory for what you may have done to cause this. Sometimes it's easier blame yourself; if you could just find a reason, you might be able to prevent this from happening to you again.

Loss of a fetus almost invariably occurs for reasons beyond the mother's control. The great majority of losses are caused by fetal chromosomal abnormalities. This does not mean that you or your partner have a genetic problem; it just means that at the moment of conception, something went wrong. The risk of chromosomal abnormalities increases as a woman gets older. Less common causes of fetal loss include infection, clotting abnormalities, and variations in the anatomy of the uterus. Later losses may be caused by cervical incompetence (a weakening of the structure of the cervix), preterm labor, or preterm rupture of the membranes, all of which may lead to premature birth. Loss in the third trimester may be related to complications such as preeclampsia, placenta previa (the placenta covers or is close to the opening of the cervix), or placental abruption (the placenta separates from the wall of the uterus).

Healing from a pregnancy loss is a physical, emotional, and spiritual process. There are, however, a few traditional Jewish rituals that will help you through this process. The traditional Jewish practice for the mother after a miscarriage or pregnancy loss is to go to the *mikvah*, the ritual bath. Jewish rituals of mourning—a funeral, sitting *shiva*, reciting the kaddish—are not practiced after a miscarriage. In the case of a stillbirth, a name is given to the baby and, for boys, circumcision may be performed. Traditionally, mourning rituals are only done for a baby that has lived at least thirty days, but the Conservative and Reform movements allow for full mourning rites if the family desires it for babies who do not live one month.

More recently, in response to the needs of women who have suffered from pregnancy loss, public and private rituals have been developed. Many helpful prayers and rituals can be found in the book *Tears of Sorrow, Seeds of Hope: A Jewish Spiritual Companion for Infertility and Pregnancy Loss* (Jewish Lights) by Nina Beth Cardin and at www.ritualwell.org, a website of Jewish feminist rituals.

We encourage you to mourn in the way that is most comforting to you, whether you work through your grief solely with your partner, or whether you choose to seek support from family, friends, or your community. If you do wish to use a public ritual to mark this event, we have included the following prayers. They are to be recited with *Birkat Hagomel*, the prayer said during the reading of the Torah by someone who has survived a difficult journey or illness (see p. 98 for a full description of this custom).

A Synagogue Ritual for Miscarriage[2]

[Woman or rabbi recites:]

Out of the depths I call to You, O God; You hear me fully when I call. God is with me, I have no fear. I was hard-pressed, about to fall; God came to my help. God, You are my strength and my courage. I will not die, but live, and yet tell of the deeds of God. I thank You for having heard me; O God, be my deliverance.

[Woman recites Birkat Hagomel*]*

בָּרוּךְ אַתָּה יְיָ אֱלֹהֵינוּ מֶלֶךְ הָעוֹלָם, הַגּוֹמֵל לְחַיָּבִים טוֹבוֹת, שֶׁגְּמָלַנִי כָּל טוֹב.

Barukh atah Adonai eloheinu melekh ha'olam, hagomel lechayavim tovot, shegemalani kol tov.

Blessed are You, Adonai our God, ruler of the universe, showing goodness to us beyond our merits, for bestowing favor upon me.

[Congregation responds:]

מִי שֶׁגְּמָלֵךְ כָּל טוֹב, הִיא תִגְמְלֵךְ כָּל טוֹב. סֶלָה. אָמֵן.

Mi shegemalekh kol tov, he yigmalekh kol tov. Selah. Amen.

May the One who has shown you every kindness, ever show kindness to you. *Selah.* **Amen.**

The rabbi may offer the following *mi shebeirakh*, a special prayer of comfort and healing for the couple:

May God who blessed our ancestors, Abraham, Isaac, and Jacob, Sarah, Rebekah, Rachel, and Leah, grant this family *refu'at hanefesh urefu'at haguf*, a full healing of body and spirit, abundant blessings from loved ones, and an awareness of

God's presence with them in their pain. As for the baby that was not to be, shelter this spirit, O God, in the shadow of Your wings, for You, God of parents, God of children, God of us all, guard and shelter us. You are a gracious and loving God. Guard our coming and our going, grant us life and peace, now and always, for You are the Source of life and peace. May we as a holy community support and love our friends in times of pain as well as times of joy. And as we have wept together, so may we soon gather to rejoice. Amen.

[In response, the woman or the couple may say:]

God heals the broken-hearted
and binds up their wounds.
God reckons the number of stars,
giving each one its name.
Great is God and full of power
whose wisdom is beyond reckoning.
God gives courage to the lowly
and brings hope to those bereft.
So may God always be with us.

—Based on Psalm 147:2–6

We also offer the following two-part poem, alternatively comforting and defiant, forgiving of God and angry at the One who gives and takes away.

One Hundred and Eighty Degrees:
A Miscarriage

I called to You God, and You answered
With joy I looked at the positive pregnancy test
For weeks and months I felt a new connection
My body changed
My lips whispered plans

We became more than
We, two
I waited, I hoped

I spoke to my little new potential
I watched for signs, for movement
Did you answer, I thought you did

I smelled blood
And then I saw it
Still convinced that you were with me
But you weren't

I call to God from this narrow place
Answer me
With your face, not your back
Heal my body
Soothe my anger against You

I forgive my body and my God
I move through the days, the months
My lips whisper prayers, hopes

∽

I'm not on speaking terms with God
Not since the miscarriage, that is
I mean, would you be?

The day of the positive pregnancy test was so wonderful
I know, you're supposed to realize
OK, miscarriage is really common
But, I wasn't going to be the one

Sometimes I wonder if it's viral
It's really going around
Everyone I know has had one

In the weeks and months when I was pregnant
I spoke to my new little potential
Hang in there, *motek,* I said
I guess it didn't help

And I was nauseous as hell,
I even complained about it
Imagine

Then I smelled the blood
Spotting
The radiologist said she was so sorry, said she had been there

One hundred and eighty degrees,
I just wanted that thing out of me
And I was still nauseous

Procedures and drugs and
Now I'm not pregnant anymore
Why me?
Do I deserve to be punished?

I'm taking care of me now
I'm healing, sometimes reluctantly
God can keep calling, I may answer
Tomorrow

—Sandy Falk

Aleph-Bet Yoga for Pregnancy

Steven A. Rapp

Yoga for Overall Well-Being during Pregnancy

Unlike almost any other time in your life, you have the unique opportunity during pregnancy to make a difference in your health as well as someone else's. Although there are many health risk factors that you cannot easily control, you can control what you eat and drink; how much fresh air, exercise, and sleep you get; and how much time you set aside for quiet activities. These represent opportunities for you to make choices that can have a positive effect on you and your growing baby's well-being. Even if you have been living a healthy lifestyle before getting pregnant, this is an ideal time to take a fresh look at your routine and consider any adjustments that might be appropriate now that you are carrying a developing child within you. For example, if you have been keeping fit through high-impact exercise, such as running or step-aerobics, you may want to consider other lower impact alternatives for this special time. Similarly, if you have not been exercising regularly, you may want to start a program that is challenging enough to make you stronger yet gentle enough for you to continue throughout your pregnancy and beyond.

Yoga is an excellent choice in either case. Yoga is gentle enough for you to practice safely every day, yet challenging enough for you to build strength and endurance. In recent years, yoga has become very popular precisely because it offers anyone, regardless of age or physical condition, a system of caring for overall health. During pregnancy, yoga can be especially beneficial to you and your unborn child because it also includes a contemplative aspect that helps you maintain your emotional balance during a period of intense physiological change. Whether you are familiar with yoga already or are just beginning, I hope that you will use the following chapter to enhance and enrich your pregnancy.

What is yoga?

Yoga is a systematic method of learning to improve your body, mind, and spirit in order to realize your true potential. Although yoga is not a religion, it complements any religious tradition by providing you with a means of connecting with the Divine Spirit within. This chapter introduces you to Aleph-Bet Yoga, a way of approaching a yoga practice from a Jewish orientation.

There are four main paths to yoga: the yoga of action, the yoga of devotion, the yoga of knowledge, and the yoga of physical and mental control. This last type of yoga is known as *raja*, or royal yoga; this is what most Westerners think of as yoga. A special branch of raja yoga is called *hatha yoga*. Hatha yoga teaches mastery of the body and control of the breath. Hatha yoga uses poses, or *asanas*, that often mimic animals or forces found in the natural world. Moving the body into and holding asanas exercises and massages all parts of the body. Many of the basic hatha yoga movements, such as bending to touch your toes, are similar to stretching exercises used by gymnasts, dancers, and athletes, but they differ in the length of time the positions are held as well as in how they are linked together to form a sequence.

Hatha yoga can be practiced as a form of physical exercise, but, when practiced with the proper intention, it can be much more than that. Although hatha yoga is primarily a system of movements that tone the whole body, the contemplative movements and breathing techniques also focus the mind for spiritual or meditative endeavors. Hatha yoga helps you improve your mental focus and balance, allowing you to apply yourself fully to all other facets of your life.

Why practice yoga during pregnancy?

Although I have never been pregnant or given birth, I have been practicing and teaching yoga for many years and have seen the enormous difference yoga has made in my wife's (three!) and friends' pregnancies, deliveries, and recoveries. Yoga is beneficial to your health and well-being at any time in your life, but it is particularly helpful for a woman who is expecting to give or has recently given birth. The combination of stretching, strengthening, breathing, and relaxation exercises involved in hatha yoga is ideal for preparing a woman for one of the most challenging events in her life. Practicing yoga during pregnancy can make your pregnancy and delivery more comfortable, healthier, and less stressful. Practicing yoga during and after your pregnancy will also give you more energy, make you stronger, and help you look your best. Even if you have never tried yoga before, perhaps because you have felt inflexible or intimidated by advanced positions you have seen in photos or on TV, please do not be intimidated. The yoga presented in this book is geared to beginners, and you will begin to realize yoga's benefits as soon as you begin.

A regular yoga practice creates a feeling of overall well-being. It helps you regain lost flexibility, improves posture, and lessens or eliminates minor aches and pains. Yoga helps counteract long hours spent sitting in chairs. It relieves the muscle stiffness and soreness that often accompany a pregnancy or physical exertion. Yoga postures massage the internal organs and glandular systems, helping regulate and optimize hormone levels, appetite, and blood circulation—particularly important during the rapid changes your body goes through during pregnancy. Yoga increases blood flow to the brain, improving concentration and memory. Equally as important, yoga helps you let go of physical and emotional tension, deepens self-awareness, and increases intuition.

Although regularly practicing yoga improves your flexibility, hatha yoga includes many poses that strengthen all the muscle groups in the body as well. Many hatha yoga poses require holding one pose, or asana, for up to several minutes, using gravity and the weight of the body to build strength. Practicing yoga strengthens the legs, hips, abdomen, and lower back, which are particularly important to a healthy pregnancy and delivery. Similarly, after delivery, practicing yoga helps rebuild your strength and speed your body's recovery.

Another benefit of practicing yoga during pregnancy is relaxation. During this period of intense change in your life, it is natural to feel some anxiety and mental stress. Through meditative movements and deep relaxation, yoga helps you quiet your mind, bringing a sense of peace and oneness. Hatha yoga deepens your breathing, lowers your blood pressure, and releases tension throughout the body. The meditative movements of slowly getting into and holding each of the poses help improve concentration. The deep, slow, steady breathing used in yoga helps the mind focus and relax simultaneously.

For which parts of the pregnant body is yoga particularly helpful?

During pregnancy, dramatic changes occur throughout your body. Most evident are the changes in the pelvic region and back. You also feel the weight of the developing child in your shoulders and neck, especially during the second and third trimesters. Practicing yoga benefits your whole body, but it is particularly helpful for stretching and strengthening these regions for an easier, more comfortable pregnancy and delivery.

For example, practicing yoga can help you gently prepare for the delivery by stretching and strengthening the area around your pelvis, including the muscles and ligaments surrounding the birth canal. After puberty, the ligaments surrounding the pelvis grow increasingly inflexible. Additionally, sitting in chairs can cause the muscles of the lower back to atrophy and weaken. During pregnancy, these imbalances can cause stiffness, discomfort, and often pain in the lower back and hip areas. Inflexibility in this region can narrow the birth canal and complicate delivery. The Aleph-Bet Yoga Series found at the end of this chapter includes a number of postures that improve flexibility of the pelvic region, broadening the potential space through which your baby will pass.

You will undoubtedly find that the added weight of the baby strains your shoulders, neck, and lower back. You may also find that your hands and wrists become swollen and stiff due to the increase in fluid that your body is retaining. Similarly, one of the unpleasant side effects of the body producing extra hormones during pregnancy is the slackening of muscles that surround tubular organs, such as the esophagus and veins. This slackening causes heartburn and swelling of the extremities, particularly the ankles, where blood tends to pool as a result of gravity. Practicing yoga can help ease all these common pregnancy symptoms by gently stretching and massaging the muscles and soft tissues.

How does yoga help with breathing during pregnancy?

Pregnancy dramatically affects your ability to breathe. As pregnancy progresses, your growing baby pushes up against your diaphragm, gradually taking up more and more of the breathing space in your lower chest. By the end of the third trimester, many women are using only the top third of their lungs to breathe and find themselves frequently out of breath after even mild exertion. Such restricted breathing reduces the amount of oxygen in your body, which can cause a mild sense of panic. Over time, shallow breathing can leave a person feeling exhausted and easily confused, angry, or depressed. Deep yoga breathing is extremely helpful in alleviating these symptoms, as it expands your breathing space along the rib cage, allowing you to breathe in more air with the space available in your chest and lungs. Deep breathing also provides your unborn baby with more oxygen, which it needs for proper growth and development.

When practicing a pose, you should try to breathe as deeply and evenly as you can through your nose, not your mouth. Do not hold your breath. Use all the space in your lungs to breathe. It is important to inhale and exhale as deeply as you can while practicing yoga, beginning by extending the diaphragm (the belly below the ribs), followed by the lower ribs, then the upper ribs. To exhale deeply, reverse the order, emptying the upper rib cage, then the lower rib cage, then the diaphragm.

Practicing the Aleph-Bet Yoga Series helps stretch and expand the rib cage and strengthens the diaphragm, which also increases the amount of air you breathe. Practicing the poses for three to five deep, even breaths for each pose increases your breathing volume and rate, providing more oxygen for you and your growing baby. With more oxygen available in your system, you will feel more energized and able to focus. The deeper breathing also relaxes your body and eases mental tension, enhancing your overall well-being.

Yoga for Each Stage of Your Pregnancy

Why practice yoga during the first trimester?

As the reality of being pregnant sinks in, the first trimester of pregnancy may be one of the most emotional and stressful periods of your life. During this period, you may feel a tremendous amount of excitement at the realization that an important journey has begun. But you may also feel a certain level of fear and anxiety as your body changes and you sense a loss of control over the process and your life. Also during the first trimester, your body is going through dramatic changes, producing about one hundred times the amount of hormones that it normally produces. Perhaps the most noticeable physical effects in the first trimester are nausea in the mornings (i.e., "morning sickness") and extreme fatigue, especially at the end of the day.

Yoga is an effective means of bringing the physical, mental, and emotional stresses of your life under control. During this time of discovery and growth, yoga can help you increase your strength and flexibility while providing you with an effective way of relaxing deeply and letting go of stress. During the first trimester, yoga can also help you center yourself and deepen your spirituality, as intense feelings begin to emerge. Practicing yoga during the first trimester can help alleviate the nausea of morning sickness through movements that provide your abdomen with a gentle massage. Because yoga should be practiced on an empty stomach, if you do have morning sickness, you might consider practicing yoga first thing in the morning, instead of eating, to wake your system gently. The deep breathing of yoga brings more oxygen into your system, and the head-to-toe stretching that yoga provides can help energize you when you feel "drained."

Why practice yoga during the second trimester?

The second trimester is an ideal time for practicing yoga. During the second trimester, your body's transformation is well on its way. Your body is still changing, but the extreme fatigue and morning sickness have likely decreased. It is often a quiet waiting period, with time to focus on what positive things you can do for yourself and your baby.

During the second trimester, practicing yoga is easier than before your pregnancy started. Your body is still producing extra hormones, which allow your muscles and connective tissues to stretch farther than before you became pregnant; this makes it easier to move into the yoga poses. In the second trimester, practicing yoga also helps you build and maintain your strength to keep you fit and feeling healthy. Additionally, practicing yoga helps you manage any stress that you may be feeling and helps you experience deep relaxation, which contributes to your overall sense of well-being.

During this time, however, you may start to feel some new physical discomforts. Your abdomen may begin to "show" and, by the end of this trimester, you may start to feel "fat." Your breasts may feel tender and begin to swell. Your wrists and ankles may feel stiff or swollen, particularly at the end of the day. Practicing yoga at this stage can help keep your whole body feeling strong and alleviate any stiffness and swelling in your breasts and extremities.

Why practice yoga during the third trimester?

During the third trimester, your body completes its physical transformation. Your baby now occupies its maximum space between your ribs and your pelvic floor. As you approach the final weeks of the pregnancy, you may grow restless for the delivery and unable to sit still as the nesting instinct kicks in. Practicing yoga in the third trimester can help you feel fit and well right through the time of delivery. Regularly practicing yoga during this trimester can also alleviate anxiety and physical discomfort and help you relax and experience an overall sense of calm and well-being.

During the third trimester, you may find that breathing has become more difficult. The deep inhaling and exhaling used in yoga can help you expand your breathing and bring the maximum amount of oxygen into your body and to your developing baby. Similarly, during this time, your lower back may ache and your breasts may become even more sensitive. Yoga will stretch, strengthen, and massage your lower back as well as the tissue surrounding and supporting your breasts. You may have discomfort and swelling in your hands, wrists, feet, and ankles as your body "softens" to prepare for the birth. Yoga stretches and gently massages your feet and ankles and helps reduce the swelling around your wrists and hands.

Why practice yoga after delivery?

Practicing yoga is an excellent method of recovering your "self" after pregnancy and delivery. The delivery of your baby marks the end of one period of your life and the beginning of another. The delivery is also a traumatic experience for your body. Practicing yoga after the delivery can help you recover your strength, realign your spine, and relieve some of the anxiety of caring for a newborn child.

Physically, practicing yoga postures tones and realigns the parts of your body that have been stretched during the pregnancy and delivery. It helps flatten your abdomen and firms the muscles around your pelvis. Practicing yoga stretches and realigns your spine and neck, which have been carrying much of the extra weight of your baby during the pregnancy. Mentally and spiritually, practicing yoga regularly following the birth provides you with a quiet, meditative time for yourself during a period that may otherwise feel as if you are absorbed totally by the needs of your baby.

Why should fathers/fathers-to-be practice yoga too?

Practicing yoga offers many benefits to mothers-to-be, and it has a lot to offer dads, too. Yoga has helped me and many other fathers-to-be/new fathers remain calmer, stay more flexible (physically and mentally), and avoid gaining sympathy weight as we played our supporting roles throughout the pregnancy and after delivery. Fathers-to-be often feel that they are not a direct part of the pregnancy process, particularly due to their lack of a physical connection to the baby's development. But rather than sitting on the physical sidelines, I recommend that fathers-to-be practice the yoga in this book with their pregnant partners as a means of getting integrally involved in enhancing the well-being of mother, father, and baby.

Yoga for the Jewish Soul

Does prenatal yoga include a spiritual component?

Beyond the physical benefits, yoga is also an excellent method for helping a woman prepare spiritually and emotionally for the enormous life changes that take place during and after pregnancy.

Pregnancy represents a unique period that can be physically demanding but also deeply spiritual, presenting many of life's deepest mysteries squarely in a woman's lap. Practicing yoga gently increases your self-awareness and gives you the opportunity for regular self-reflection. Through its slow meditative movements, deep breathing, and steady concentrated effort, yoga practice can help you modulate your emotions, increase your compassion, and open your mind to spiritual experiences and feelings. In this way, practicing yoga can awaken your body's inherent psychospiritual energy, or *kundalini*, which is said to rise through energy centers, or *chakras*, along the spine. This awakening of the energy centers is remarkably similar to the movement of spiritual energy through the body's *sefirot* described in the Jewish mystical writings of Kabbalah. Many people who begin to practice yoga for the physical benefits are surprised when this subtle awakening creates new interest in deepening their spiritual practice, such as through prayer, study, or selfless service (what many Jews call "*mitzvah* work," or *tikkun olam*, repairing the world).

How can yoga be Jewish?

It has often been said that yoga without spirituality is just gymnastics. This means that in order to realize the full potential of yoga practice, the physical exercises must be complemented with some form of spiritual effort. Many Jewish people practice yoga for its physical benefits. From my experience as a Jewish yoga practitioner and teacher, I believe that a substantial number of us would also like our yoga practice to connect with our Judaism. The yoga described in this book is based on my book, *Aleph-Bet Yoga: Embodying the Hebrew Letters for Physical and Spiritual Well-Being* (Jewish Lights). Aleph-Bet Yoga provides a way for Jews and others to include a meaningful spiritual element in their yoga practice. I hope that practicing Aleph-Bet Yoga while you are pregnant, as well as long after your baby is born, will help you deepen your spiritual connection to Judaism while enhancing your sense of well-being.

The Jewish connection in Aleph-Bet Yoga is created in two basic ways. First, on a physical level, Aleph-Bet Yoga associates all twenty-seven Hebrew letters (the twenty-two regular Hebrew letters plus the five final letters for *kaf, mem, nun, pey,* and *tzadi*) with hatha yoga poses that approximate the shapes of the letters. Aleph-Bet Yoga also connects two of the thirteen Hebrew vowels, *kamatz* and *patach,* to two yoga poses that are important to do at the close of each yoga session. As a whole-body physical activity, Aleph Bet Yoga connects your body with the Hebrew letters in a way that intellectually reading or writing Hebrew normally does not.

Second, on a spiritual level, Aleph-Bet Yoga combines a Jewish intention, *kavvana,* with the physical effort of caring for our bodies through hatha yoga. To help bring this *kavvana* into your yoga practice, I include a focus/meditation along with instructions for practicing each letter-pose. The suggested meditations are based on the historical meanings of the Hebrew letters as they have come to me through Rabbi David A. Cooper's book, *Renewing Your Soul: A Guided Retreat for the Sabbath and Other Days of Rest.* For example, the Hebrew letter *dalet* symbolizes a doorway. While practicing the yoga pose associated with *dalet* (the half-forward bend), I suggest contemplating your role as the doorway to new life.

The Hebrew letters have always played a profound role in Judaism. Hebrew has been the language of the Jewish people since ancient times, and during the Diaspora it was reserved for prayers and sacred writings as a way of sanctifying them. In the Jewish mystical tradition of Kabbalah, the Hebrew letters are believed to be vessels carrying divine light. In mainstream Jewish practice, the Hebrew letters are still considered sacred because of their role in communicating God's word to humankind.

How can Aleph-Bet Yoga enhance the spiritual dimension of pregnancy?

As you begin to realize your role as the carrier of a new life, you may sense a growing connectedness to the Creator of All Life. You may find that as your baby begins to stir within you, you experience intense spiritual feelings of wonder and awe. These feelings may fill you with wonder about the miracles of pregnancy, motherhood, and your connection to the Source of All Life. Practicing Aleph-Bet Yoga can enhance the spiritual experience of your pregnancy by providing you with a way to explore those spiritual feelings in a Jewish context.

As you are practicing the poses, try to concentrate on the shape and meaning of each Hebrew letter. Contemplate the divine energy in that shape. Focus on a Hebrew word or phrase containing the letter. Meditate on the connection between your body and the shape of the letter. Imagine that your developing child is a sacred *dagesh,* or emphasis mark, within each letter you form. Before practicing a pose, read the suggested focus/meditation to yourself. Repeat it while you practice the pose. With each deep breath, try chanting the name of the letter or a name of God that contains that letter. Or contemplate a poem, a prayer, or a verse of scripture that comes to mind, such as those found throughout this book.

Simply setting aside a regular time and place to practice Aleph-Bet Yoga can also help you connect with your spiritual thoughts and feelings. Practicing Aleph-Bet Yoga with spiritual meditations daily or at least twice a week will give you a predictable opportunity for working on your spiritual practice as well as your body. Although I have included a suggested meditation to focus on while practicing each letter pose, use your imagination and your personal insights to create your own body-spirit connection with the Hebrew letters that form the words of our prayers, stories, and songs celebrating life. The important thing is to try to elevate your thoughts and create a spiritual intention that complements the physical activity you are doing. Find a spiritual approach that resonates with you, and try to work with it during your yoga practice.

For the first few months after delivery, you may feel as if your life is controlled by the demands of your baby. You may feel as if you have no time in your life for stepping back and appreciating the wonder of the experience. Regularly practicing Aleph-Bet Yoga can help you maintain a space in your life for connecting with your spiritual thoughts and feelings.

As you practice the Aleph-Bet Yoga poses after delivery, reflect on the miracle and wonder of the entire pregnancy and delivery process. Read the focus/meditation for each pose and consider whether the meaning has changed for you from the time of pregnancy to the time after delivery. Try to practice the poses with great care, with slow transitions into and out of the poses. As you form the letters with your body, allow yourself to be amazed at the changes our bodies can make. In your own way, give thanks to the Creator of the human body for its ability to change and heal.

Getting Ready to Practice

What do you need to practice yoga?

One of the inherent beauties of hatha yoga is its simplicity. Basically, all you need to practice yoga is your body and a clean, comfortable place. A hardwood floor or firm carpet gives your feet a good grip to do the standing and balancing poses. However, for seated or lying poses, a blanket, towel, or thin rug can provide a degree of hygiene and comfort. A thin (¹/₄-inch) exercise mat, known in yoga circles as a "sticky mat," works best for both the standing and the seated or lying postures. Additionally, as your pregnancy progresses into the second and third trimesters, it will be helpful to support yourself with a few simple props, such as a folded blanket, pillows, a flexible strap (an old belt or necktie works well), a sturdy chair, and a wooden or foam block (measuring approximately 9 x 4 x 3 inches).

In choosing a place to practice, look for a space where you will not be interrupted or distracted. You may choose to listen to soft music while practicing. Personally, I find it easier to "listen" to how my body feels and to focus on the letters when it is quiet. But some people find that music enhances their sense of focus and relaxation and allows them to enjoy their practice more.

Is there a benefit to taking a yoga class?

While you are trying to learn about yoga through books (and perhaps videos), I strongly recommend that you take a regular (weekly) hatha yoga class at your nearest yoga center, Jewish Community Center, or fitness center. There is no comparison between trying to teach yourself and having an experienced teacher to guide, inspire, and correct you.

Please note, however, that there are many styles of hatha yoga classes offered today and not all are suited for pregnant women or brand-new moms. For example, while you are pregnant and during the period of recovery following the delivery, I do not recommend that you take classes in the "power" yoga styles, such as Ashtanga, or "hot" yoga styles, such as Bikram. I strongly recommend that you speak with the instructor before signing up to ensure that the class is suitable for pregnancy. Many yoga centers and gyms offer special pre- and postnatal yoga classes for women. These classes are excellent because they are tailored to your body's current needs. They also provide an opportunity to meet other expectant mothers, which can give you the motivation and support you need to stick with a regular yoga practice. Some facilities even offer yoga classes for mothers and babies together, although many women I know look forward to their yoga class as a time for themselves without their babies, particularly during the chaos of the first six months following delivery.

To maintain your Jewish perspective while taking group classes, think of the Hebrew letters whenever the class does one of the corresponding poses. Alternatively, you could reflect on one of the poems or prayers in this book when you relax at the close of the session. Although the instructor may decide which poses the group works on, you can choose the focus of your inner reflection.

How to Practice the Aleph-Bet Yoga Series

For maximum benefit, you should practice regularly. As with any skill, the more you practice, the better you will get. And as with any skill, it is better to practice a short time each day rather than once a week for a long time. Ideally, you should practice long enough to hold each pose for three to five breaths (approximately 15 to 30 seconds), and then rest in between poses for 5 to 10 seconds. If you are just beginning, you may want to try the pose once, rest, and then try it again. For asymmetrical poses (poses that stretch one side differently than the other), such as *aleph* (extended triangle pose) and *chet* (half-moon pose), you should practice on one side, then the other. For maximum benefit, if your time and schedule permit, you should practice all the poses in the series every day (approximately 30 to 45 minutes). As a start, however, twice a week is probably manageable for most people. At the end of this chapter, I include guidelines for an abbreviated session (approximately 20 minutes). Try to find days and times that work for you and stick with your routine.

As you begin practicing, please try not to be judgmental with yourself. Try to relax. Yoga is not an all-or-nothing activity; the benefits come from making the effort rather than from doing each pose perfectly. Do not be discouraged if you cannot finish the pose exactly as is described the first, second, or even twentieth time you try it. Anger and frustration will only tighten your muscles. The precise forms come with time. Practicing in sight of a mirror can help you keep your spine, legs, and shoulders aligned. Rest assured that you will start to get the benefits of hatha yoga as soon as you begin trying to make the forms, no matter how imperfectly.

As you continue practicing the poses over time, you may find that you experience some unexpected or uncomfortable emotions as well. Particularly during pregnancy and the postpartum period, when your hormone levels may swing wildly, your emotions may range from the extremes of laughter to anger or sadness. This is natural. Yoga increases our awareness of where in our bodies we are stuck physically; this can also be related to emotional or psychological trauma, such as an old injury or loss. Notice the stuck spots, and use your breath to move through the resistance. Welcome any emotions and let them go. See their surfacing and release as a natural part of the healing process.

Is there a special order for practicing the poses of Aleph-Bet Yoga?

When practicing hatha yoga poses, it is important to proceed in an ordered sequence. There are hundreds of hatha yoga poses requiring varying levels of ability. Each pose stretches a targeted group of muscles and tissues. To avoid injuring yourself, or creating a structural imbalance from overstretching one side of the body, it is important that you follow a set order. Typically, a hatha yoga sequence works the outer extremities, such as the arms and legs, first, and then the core of the body, including the abdomen and spine. The poses are grouped into general categories. A common sequence for beginners starts with standing poses, then moves to sitting poses, inverted poses, lying poses, back-bends, twists, and finally a lying relaxation, with some poses falling into more than one category at the same time. Basically, this book follows this beginner's sequence.

Although this chapter describes hatha yoga poses in the order of the Hebrew *aleph-bet* (that is, in *aleph*betical order), please note that you should *not* practice the poses in that order. Rather, at the end of this chapter, you will find a table containing the series of poses that correlates to the proper sequence of a yoga session, what I call the "Aleph-Bet Yoga Series." The table indicates which poses are appropriate for the first, second, and third trimesters, as well as the recovery period following delivery. If you do not have time to do the entire series, you may choose to focus on just a few letter poses. Or you may skip some poses that are similar within each of the categories, as noted in the suggestions for shorter sessions at the end of this chapter.

How can you modify the poses as your body changes during pregnancy?

Your body will be changing dramatically over the course of your pregnancy. Some poses will need to be adjusted to accommodate these changes. To help you adapt your practice as your pregnancy proceeds, I include suggestions for modifications using simple props. For example, as your pregnancy progresses into the second and third trimesters, it is helpful to support yourself with a few simple props, as described earlier. You may find that a blanket placed beneath your buttocks relieves strain on your lower back. Similarly, you can use a strap or belt to extend your reach in seated forward-bending poses. As your center of gravity changes, using a block, wall, or chair as a hand support is helpful. For sitting and lying poses, a stack of pillows under your lower back, knees, or abdomen can provide support while allowing you to achieve the full benefits of the poses.

Cautionary Notes for Practicing Yoga during Pregnancy

Practicing yoga for most pregnant women is safe. However, *before starting or continuing a yoga practice while pregnant, you should consult with your physician. Particularly if you have a history of miscarriages or other fertility disorders or any preexisting conditions, such as high blood pressure or arthritis, your doctor may tell you to avoid certain movements or positions during certain stages of your pregnancy. You should immediately consult a doctor if you feel a sharp pain, such as in a joint, during or after practicing hatha yoga.*

Generally, whether or not you have been practicing yoga prior to your pregnancy, practicing the poses of the Aleph-Bet Yoga Series should be beneficial to you. However, some poses should be avoided during particular stages of pregnancy, as discussed in the following sections.

What poses should be avoided during the first trimester and the first two months after delivery?

At this delicate time in the pregnancy or during the recovery, you must be careful not to compress your uterus. *During the first trimester and the first two months following delivery, you should avoid practicing the following Aleph-Bet Yoga poses:* tet *(half-boat pose),* tzadi *(upright extended foot pose), final* tzadi *(extended hand to foot pose), final* mem *(forward bend pose),* ayin *(leg extension pose), and* kamatz *(stomach turning pose).*

What poses should be avoided during the second and third trimesters?

In the second trimester, your baby has completely formed and the placenta should now be secure inside your uterus, making it safe to practice the majority of the poses in the Aleph-Bet Yoga Series (with some modifications and props). By the third trimester, your body's shape has changed considerably. Most important, your center of gravity has shifted, and you may have to relearn how to balance in many of the poses. Additionally, because of the extra weight that you are carrying in the front of your body, you must take extra care not to strain your lower back while practicing. *As your pregnancy progresses to its final stages, you should consult your physician about any limitations on your activity.*

During the second and third trimesters, you should avoid or modify poses where you lie on your belly or raise your legs. *During this time, you should avoid two poses:* samech *(bow pose) and* shin *(inverted-boat pose), in which you lie directly on your stomach.* However, these poses can be practiced safely while lying on your side.

Although your belly may touch the floor in the pose for *kuf* (child's pose), you can still practice the pose safely during the second trimester by using a large pillow or seat cushion placed under your chest and head. When practicing the poses where you lift your legs, namely *tet* (boat pose) and *tzadi* (upright extended foot pose), you should bend your knees to avoid straining your back. Similarly, in your third trimester, you may find it difficult to lie flat on your back with your legs extended in *patach* (corpse pose). To avoid straining your back, either bend your knees (with a pillow under them) or roll onto your side in order to relax completely.

What other general cautions should be followed for a safe yoga practice?

Regardless of the particular trimester you are in, there are a number of general cautions you should follow as well. If you have high blood pressure, a detached retina, or an ear infection, you should always avoid inverted poses, such as *tzadi* (upright extended foot pose). If you suffer from a herniated or slipped disk, do not attempt the back-bending poses, such as final *pey* (standing back-bend), *pey* (a camel pose variation), *mem* (a camel pose variation), *shin* (inverted-boat pose), or *samech* (bow pose). If you have ever strained your back, you should be extra careful to bend your knees while practicing *tet* (half-boat pose), *tzadi* (upright extended foot pose), and *patach* (corpse pose).

Additionally, when practicing yoga, it is important to pay attention to the signals you are getting from your body. Yoga can make your body feel great, but it is also normal and okay to feel some discomfort when trying to stretch muscles and connective tissue that have not been stretched for a while (or ever). It is common to experience some unfamiliar physical sensations in some of the more challenging poses. You should always move into and out of the poses slowly and with care. Gently make adjustments to your body in each stretch. Breathe deeply and slowly through your nose. Do not bounce while stretching. Try to focus on your breathing instead of dwelling on discomfort or your distance from the ideal pose. However, you should stop and not continue a pose if you experience sharp pain or excessive tightness.

Yoga has myriad health benefits, but it is always possible to injure yourself if you are not careful or do not follow the instructions correctly. Remember to listen to your body's own wisdom about how far to push yourself. We all have our limits, and these must be respected. Do not compare yourself to others or try something that does not feel right to you. If you feel tightness in a muscle, do not fight it. Instead, use your breath to help you release the tension. Inhale until you start to feel tightness, then use your exhalation to stretch gently.

If you have any physical limitations or preexisting medical conditions, or believe you may be pregnant, consult with a physician before attempting the following postures on your own. Neither the publisher nor the author are responsible for injuries sustained from practicing the yoga poses described in this book.

The Proper Order of a Yoga Session

This chapter introduces the letters and yoga poses in the order of the Hebrew *aleph-bet* (i.e., in *aleph*betical order). However, we do not recommend that you practice the poses in this order. Rather, in the chart beginning on page 160, we have outlined a series of poses that correlate to the best order for the poses in each stage of pregnancy.

Benefits: This standing pose stretches and strengthens the feet, knees, and spine, and promotes better posture.

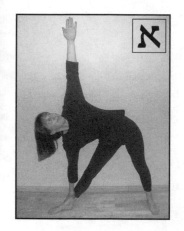

Aleph—This letter is a symbol for oxen. A corresponding yoga pose is *utthita trikonasana*, extended triangle pose.

Focus/Meditation: As the oxen labor in the field so that others can eat and live, I carry and labor with child so that future generations may live.

How to practice the pose:

1. Stand straight with your feet together and your arms by your sides. Inhale.

2. Exhale as you walk your feet apart about 4 feet, and raise your arms out to your sides, parallel to the floor, palms facing downward.

3. Keeping your hips facing forward, turn your right foot 90 degrees from the left so that the heel of your right foot is in line with the arch of your left foot. Press into the outer edges (the little toe side) of your feet.

4. Inhale and stand up as tall as you can, lengthening your spine. Keep both your arms and your legs straight and, as you exhale, reach to the right as far as you can with your right hand, as if you were reaching for a rescue line, making sure your feet are stuck to the floor. Keeping your spine long, lower your straight right arm and hand to wherever it touches your straight right leg and raise your straight left arm so that it is pointing straight up. Try not to put pressure on your right hand.

5. Inhale and turn your head and try to look up at your left hand. If this feels like too much of a stretch for your neck, just turn your head to face horizontally.

6. Smile and take three to five deep breaths (15 to 30 seconds), releasing any tension you feel in your hamstrings or lower back with each exhalation.

7. Inhale while reaching up toward the ceiling with your left hand. Bring your torso back to center with your arms parallel to the floor.

8. Switch the position of your feet and do steps 3 through 6 on the left side.

9. Walk your feet back together and bring your arms back down to your sides.

Variations: During the **second trimester,** you can modify the pose by simply moving the bottom hand higher up the forward leg, resting your hand above your knee or on your thigh, or resting your hand on a block by your foot. During the **third trimester,** you can modify the pose by bending the forward knee slightly as you bring your hand down to rest on your thigh or knee. Alternatively, you can rest your lower hand on a chair.

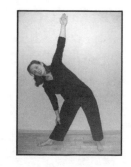

Benefits: This standing pose stretches and strengthens the feet, ankles, and knees; aligns the spine for better posture; strengthens the arms and shoulders; and reduces swelling in the ankles and feet.

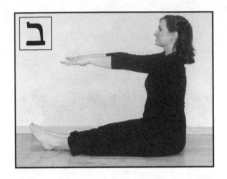

Bet—This letter is a symbol for a house. A corresponding yoga pose is a variation of *dandasana*, stick pose with arms extended, and *pawanmuktasana*, "wind releasing" series for the feet and ankles.

Focus/Meditation: My body is a living tabernacle, a temple of my soul and new life.

How to practice the pose:

1. Sit on the floor with your legs together and extended straight out.

2. Flex your feet so your toes point back toward your body.

3. Inhale and sit up as straight as possible, lifting your rib cage and chin. Straighten your spine as if there were a string running through your spine, through your head, and someone were pulling it up.

4. Exhale and straighten your arms in front of you so they are parallel to the floor. Reach straight ahead through your fingertips but keep your back straight.

Do not bend forward.

5. Smile and take three to five deep breaths.

6. Lower your arms. Shake your legs gently.

7. Now, with your knees straight, inhale and point your toes to the ceiling (flexing the toes). Exhale and point them forward (pointing the toes). Repeat this flexing and pointing three times.

8. With your knees still straight, rotate your feet three times to the left and then three times to the right, making the biggest circles you can.

Variations: During the **second trimester,** you can modify the pose by placing a cushion or pillow under your buttocks.

During the **third trimester,** you can modify the pose by sitting with your back flat against a wall or sturdy piece of furniture, and with a pillow or cushion under your buttocks.

Benefits: This standing pose stretches and strengthens the groin muscles, knees, hips, spine, shoulders, and neck; expands breathing capacity; warms the body; and improves circulation.

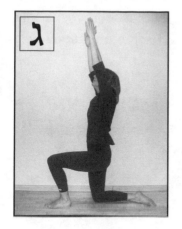

Gimmel—This letter is a symbol for a camel. A corresponding yoga pose is a variation of *virabhadrasana*, warrior I pose.

Focus/Meditation: Strength of Israel, help me carry, deliver, and care for this child.

How to practice the pose:

1. Stand straight with your feet together and your arms by your sides. Inhale.

2. Exhale as you walk your feet apart 4 feet with both feet pointing forward.

3. Inhale and raise your arms straight up in the air and reach up as high as you can. Look up between your hands.

4. Turn your right foot 90 degrees so that your right heel is in line with the arch of your left foot.

5. While still stretching upward with your arms, exhale and rotate your hips to face right (the same direction as your right foot is pointing).

6. Come on to the ball of your left foot, and bend your right knee 90 degrees as you drop your left knee to the floor. For a deeper stretch, keep your left leg straight and your left foot flat on the floor.

7. Smile and take three to five deep breaths.

8. Inhale and straighten your legs. Rotate your hips back to center.

9. Exhale and lower your arms.

10. Repeat steps 3 through 8 on the other side.

11. Walk your feet back together.

Variations: During the **second trimester,** you can modify the pose by placing a cushion under your knee that is touching the floor.

During the **third trimester,** you can modify the pose by placing a cushion under the knee on the floor and a chair under your pelvis so that your weight is supported.

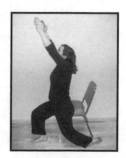

Benefits: This standing pose stretches and strengthens the arms, shoulders, lower back, stomach, legs, and feet; helps digestion; and calms the mind.

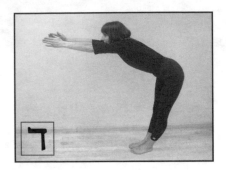

Dalet—This letter is a symbol of a doorway. A corresponding yoga pose is a variation on *uttanasana*, forward extension pose.

Focus/Meditation: *El Shaddai*, bless me, for I am a doorway to the world through which new life will pass.

How to practice the pose:

1. Stand up as straight as possible with your feet together and your arms by your side. Inhale and lift your rib cage and chin. Exhale.

2. Inhale and raise your arms as high as possible. Really stretch your hands toward the ceiling. Look up between your hands.

3. Exhale and slowly reach forward, bending at the hips and lowering your arms and back in one straight line until your upper body is parallel to the floor. Keep looking forward through your hands.

4. Smile and take three to five deep breaths.

5. On the last exhale, lower your arms and back as far down as possible.

6. On the next inhale, slowly raise your upper body, reaching up with your arms.

7. Exhale and lower your arms.

Variations: During the **second trimester,** you can modify the pose by holding on to a windowsill or the back of a chair for support.

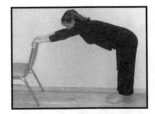

During the **third trimester,** you can modify the pose by facing a wall at a distance of 2 feet. Raise your arms as high as you can and place them on the wall. Walking slowly backward, walk your hands down the wall as far as you feel comfortable.

Benefits: This standing pose stretches and strengthens the feet, ankles, legs, hips, and lower back; lengthens the spine; and improves posture.

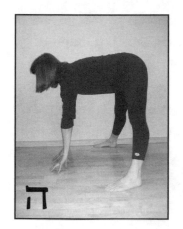

Hay—This letter is a symbol for taking. A corresponding yoga pose is *prasarita padottanasana*, extended foot pose.

Focus/Meditation: *Eloheinu,* may every breath my child takes be full of praise and appreciation for the wonders of creation.

How to practice the pose:

1. Stand up as straight as possible with your arms by your side. Inhale.

2. Exhale as you walk your feet apart 4 feet and place your hands on your hips.

3. Inhale as you raise your hands above your head.

4. Exhale as you bend at the waist until your upper body is parallel to the floor.

5. Place both hands on the floor, touching with your fingertips or palms. Keep your head and neck straight, looking down at the floor without bending your neck.

6. Smile and take three to five deep breaths.

7. Place your hands on your hips. Inhale and slowly lift your upper body back up to a standing position.

8. Exhale and walk your feet back together.

Variations: During the **second trimester,** you may want to modify the pose by placing a yoga block or thick book under your hands.

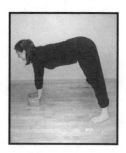

During the **third trimester,** you may want to modify the pose by placing a block or thick book under your hands and placing your head on the seat of a chair for support.

Benefits: This standing pose stretches and strengthens the feet and knees, and aligns the spine for better posture.

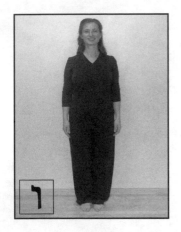

Vav—This letter means "and," and symbolizes connection. A corresponding yoga pose is *tadasana*, mountain pose.

Focus/Meditation: God, the soul You placed within me is pure. And now, temporarily, my body holds a second soul, waiting to be born.

How to practice the pose:

1. Stand with your feet together and your arms by your sides.

2. Inhale and lift your rib cage and chin.

3. Exhale and relax your shoulders. Your legs should be straight and flexed. Push down through your feet. Imagine a string running through your spine and out the crown of your head. Imagine that someone is pulling the string up so that you grow straighter and taller with each breath.

4. Smile and take three to five deep breaths.

Variations: During the **second** and **third trimesters,** you may want to modify the pose by raising your arms over your head to create more breathing space and to stretch your upper back.

Benefits: This standing pose stretches and strengthens the feet and knees; aligns the spine for better posture; and strengthens the arms and shoulders.

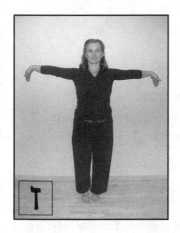

Zayin—This letter is a symbol for a weapon or to sustain. A corresponding yoga pose is the rooster, a variation on *tadasana*, mountain pose.

Focus/Meditation: Blessed are You, Adonai our God, ruler of the universe, who gives us life, sustains us, and enables us to reach this moment.

How to practice the pose:

1. Stand up as straight as possible with your arms by your sides. Inhale.

2. Exhale and raise your arms so they are parallel to the floor, fingers pointing down.

3. Inhale and roll up onto the balls of your feet. Reach upward through the crown of your head.

4. Smile and take three to five deep breaths.

5. Exhale, lower your arms, and come down onto flat feet.

Variations: During the **second** and **third trimesters,** you may want to modify the pose by holding on to a wall with one hand for more secure balance.

Benefits: This standing pose stretches and strengthens the ankles, legs, hips, lower back, and neck; lengthens the spine; promotes balance; and improves posture.

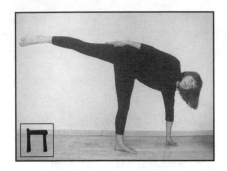

Chet—This letter is the symbol for life. A corresponding yoga pose is *ardha chandrasana*, half-moon pose.

Focus/Meditation: Source of Life, may my child grow to appreciate the miracles of everyday life.

How to practice the pose:

1. Stand straight with your feet together and your arms by your sides. Inhale.

2. Exhale and walk your feet apart 4 feet and raise your arms out to your sides, parallel to the floor, with palms facing downward.

3. Turn your left foot 90 degrees to the left so that the heel of your left foot is in line with the arch of your right foot. Your arms and legs should be straight. Your hips should be facing forward.

4. Inhale and bend your left knee as you reach your left hand down to the floor, placing the fingertips of your left hand 6 to 12 inches ahead of the toes of your left foot. Keep your right leg straight.

5. Place all your weight on your left leg. Exhale as you straighten your left leg while lifting your straight right leg completely off the floor. You should be balancing on your left foot and fingertips. Your hips should be facing forward. Make sure that your right leg is

straight and your toes are flexed strongly—this will help you balance.

7. Inhale and place your right arm on your right leg. Look straight ahead or up at the ceiling.

8. Smile and take three to five deep breaths.

9. Exhale and slowly lower your straight right leg while bending your left leg.

10. Inhale and straighten your left leg. Bring your left hand back to your left shin or wherever it comfortably reaches on your left leg. Exhale and raise your straight right arm back up pointing toward the ceiling. Both legs should now be straight. You should be back in the triangle pose (see *aleph*).

11. Inhale while reaching up through your right hand. Bring your upper body back to the center with your arms parallel to the floor.

12. Switch feet and follow steps 3 through 11 on the other side.

13. Inhale and turn both feet so they face forward, then walk your feet together. Exhale and lower your arms.

Variations: During the **second trimester,** you may want to modify the pose by resting your bottom hand on a yoga block, a large book, or a chair for easier balance and support.

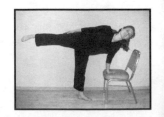

During the **third trimester,** you may want to modify the pose by placing both hands on the seat of a chair for additional support.

Benefits: This seated pose strengthens the abdomen and lower back; aids digestion; warms the body; and improves balance.

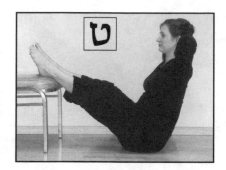

Tet—This letter is a symbol for goodness. A corresponding yoga pose is *ardha navasana*, half-boat pose.

Focus/Meditation: *Hashem Tov*, the Good Name, may my child fill its life with good deeds.

How to practice the pose:

1. Sit on the floor with your legs straight in front of you, your toes pointed forward, and your arms at your sides.

2. Sitting up straight, inhale, bring your hands behind your head, and interlace your fingers.

3. Exhale and, with a straight back, lean your upper body halfway back.

4. Simultaneously raise your straight legs together as high as you can, coming to rest on a chair or yoga block. If you have a history of back problems, you should bend your knees before you lift them.

5. Smile and take three to five deep breaths, making sure you keep your back straight and not rounded.

6. Exhale, slowly lower your legs, and sit up straight. Lower your arms.

Cautions and Variations: As previously discussed, *I do not recommend practicing this pose during the first trimester or during the first eight weeks following delivery.*

During the **third trimester,** you may want to modify the pose by bending your knees and placing stacks of pillows under your feet, knees, and behind your lower back for support.

Benefits: These movements stretch and strengthen the wrists, hands, and fingers; improve circulation; and release built-up wastes, or "wind," from the joints.

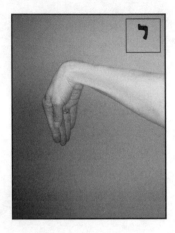

Yud—This letter is a symbol for the hand. A corresponding yoga pose is part of *pawanmuktasana*, "wind relieving" series for the hands and wrists.

Focus/Meditation: Eternal God, may my child's hands help repair the world.

How to practice the pose:

1. Stand up as straight as possible with your arms straight out in front of you.

2. Inhale as you bend your wrists so that your fingers point straight up toward the ceiling.

3. Exhale as you bend your wrists so that your fingers point down toward the floor.

4. Repeat steps 2 and 3 three times. Point your fingers up on the inhale, down on the exhale.

5. With straight arms, extend your hands with your palms facing up.

6. Inhale as you bend your wrists so that your fingers point up toward the ceiling.

7. Exhale as you open your palms and point your fingers down toward the floor.

8. Repeat steps 6 and 7 three times. Point your fingers up on the inhale, down on the exhale.

9. On the next inhale, point your fingers up toward the ceiling. As you exhale, rotate both hands to the right three times. Inhale and rotate your hands to the left three times, keeping your elbows straight and locked.

Variations: In the **second and third trimesters,** you may want to modify the pose by sitting on a chair.

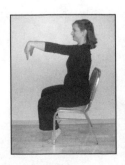

Benefits: This seated pose stretches and strengthens the thighs, knees, lower back, arms, shoulders, and neck; improves circulation; calms the mind; massages internal organs; and improves digestion.

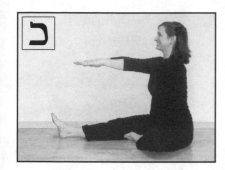

Kaf—This letter is a symbol for the palm of the hand. A corresponding yoga pose is *janu sirsasana*, knee-head pose.

Focus/Meditation: Blessed are You, Adonai our God, in whose hand is the breath of life.

How to practice the pose:

1. Sit with your legs straight out in front of you. Inhale deeply.

2. Bend your right leg and place the sole of your right foot on the inside of your left thigh. Exhale and relax as you let your right knee drop as close to the floor as is comfortable.

3. Inhale and raise your arms straight up above your head.

4. Exhale and lower your arms until they are parallel to the floor.

5. Inhale and sit up straight. Exhale and lean forward from the hips. Reach forward (horizontally) as far as you can. To avoid straining your neck, reach with your chin, rather than your forehead, toward your big toe.

6. Smile and take three to five deep breaths.

7. Inhale, sit up straight and raise your arms above your head.

8. Exhale and bring your arms down.

9. Switch legs and repeat on the other side.

Variations: During the **second** and **third trimesters,** you can modify the pose by placing a cushion under your buttocks and looping a strap around your foot to extend your reach.

Benefits: This standing pose stretches and strengthens the knees, ankles, feet, and toes; strengthens and aligns the spine; promotes better posture; and strengthens the arms and shoulders.

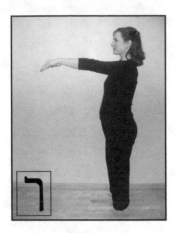

Final *Kaf*—This letter is a symbol for the palm of the hand. A corresponding yoga pose is a variation on *tadasana*, mountain pose.

Focus/Meditation: Merciful God, may my child's hands be generous and open, always ready to help those in need.

How to practice the pose:

1. Stand with your feet together and your arms by your sides.

2. Inhale and lift your rib cage and chin. Lengthen your spine.

3. Exhale and relax your shoulders. Your legs should be straight and flexed. Push down through your feet. Imagine a string running through your spine and out the crown of your head. Imagine that some-one is pulling up the string so that you grow straighter and taller with each breath.

4. Inhale and raise your arms in front of you until they are parallel to the floor. Look straight ahead.

5. Stand on your tiptoes or the balls of your feet.

6. Smile and take three to five deep breaths.

7. Exhale, lower your arms, and come down onto flat feet.

Variations: During the **second** and **third trimesters,** you may want to modify the pose by placing your hands on a wall in front of you for support.

Benefits: This standing pose stretches and strengthens the feet, ankles, knees, thighs, hips, shoulders, and spine.

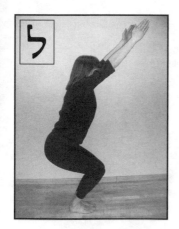

Lamed—This letter is a symbol for learning or teaching. A corresponding yoga pose is *utkatasana*, lightning pose.

Focus/Meditation: Source of Knowledge, may the child that I bear be dedicated to learning the knowledge of our people.

How to practice the pose:

1. Stand up as straight as possible with your arms by your sides.

2. Inhale and raise your arms above your head, in line with your torso and with your palms facing each other. Reach as high as you can, stretching your upper back.

3. Without losing the stretch in your upper back, exhale and bend both legs as much as you can, ideally until your thighs are parallel to the floor. For a deeper stretch, you may lean your torso forward slightly, keeping your back straight. Lean back on your heels and try to pull your chest up and back.

4. Smile and take three to five deep breaths.

5. Inhale and stand up straight.

6. Exhale and lower your arms.

Variations: During the **second trimester,** you may want to modify the pose by separating your feet so they are hip-width apart.

During the **third trimester,** you may want to modify the pose by separating your feet hip-width apart or more and by leaning against a wall for support. You may also rest your buttocks against the front of a chair seat for additional support.

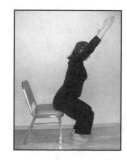

Benefits: This back-bending pose stretches and strengthens the feet, ankles, shins, knees, thighs, stomach, hips, lower back, chest, neck, arms, and hands; opens the chest and throat; energizes the whole body; and expands breathing capacity.

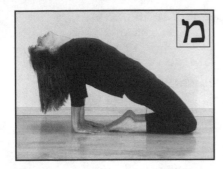

Mem—This letter is a symbol for water. A corresponding yoga pose is a variation of *ustrasana*, camel pose.

Focus/Meditation: Master of Creation, may my child be like a tree planted by a river of water, bringing forth good fruit.

How to practice the pose:

1. Kneel on both knees on the floor with your hips resting on your heels. Inhale.

2. Place both palms on the floor with your fingers facing toward your back. Exhale and lean backward.

3. Inhale and lift your hips as high as you can, tightening your buttocks.

4. Tilt your head back gently and look up at the ceiling.

5. Smile and take three to five deep breaths.

6. On the next exhale, lower your hips back down to your heels.

7. Inhale and sit up straight.

Variations: During the **second** and **third trimesters,** you can modify the pose by separating your knees hip-width apart and placing a rolled blanket between your knees and under your buttocks. To avoid straining your neck, look straight ahead and do not look at the ceiling.

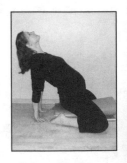

Benefits: This seated pose stretches and strengthens the thighs, knees, lower back, arms, shoulders, and neck; improves circulation; calms the mind; massages the internal organs; and improves digestion.

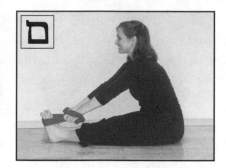

Final *Mem*—This letter is a symbol for water. A corresponding yoga pose is *paschimottanasana*, seated forward bend.

Focus/Meditation: Divine Presence, help me teach this child to sing your praises like Miriam by the sea.

How to practice the pose:

1. Sit with your legs straight out in front of you.

2. Inhale and raise your arms straight up above your head.

3. Exhale and reach your arms forward and down, using a belt or strap to loop around your feet.

4. Inhale and look up at the ceiling. Straighten your back.

5. Exhale, looking toward your toes, and reach with your chin and hands toward your feet, using the strap to pull yourself slowly forward. Try not to round your shoulders.

6. Smile and take three to five deep breaths, inching forward with your upper body with each exhale.

7. Inhale and slowly sit up straight.

Cautions and Variations: As discussed earlier, *you should not practice this pose during the first trimester or during the first eight weeks following delivery.*

During the **third trimester,** you may want to modify the pose by placing a cushion under your buttocks and placing a pillow or folded blanket on your thighs to lean on for support.

Benefits: This seated pose stretches and strengthens the ankles, knees, groin muscles, and hips; opens the hip joints for leg mobility; and strengthens and aligns the spine.

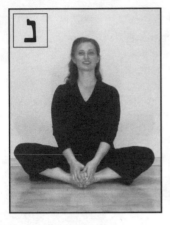 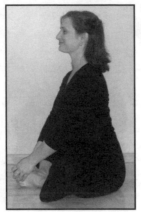

Nun—This letter is a symbol for a kingdom or a fish. A corresponding yoga pose is *badha konasana*, butterfly or cobbler pose.

Focus/Meditation:

Elohim, may this child learn to swim as swiftly as a fish.

How to practice the pose:

1. Sit with your legs straight out in front of you and inhale.

2. Exhale, bend both legs, and place the soles of your feet together.

3. Inhale, interlace your fingers, and clasp them around your toes.

4. Exhale, place your heels as close to your groin as possible, and lower your bent knees as close to the floor as is comfortable.

5. Inhale, lift your rib cage and chin, and sit up as straight as you can.

6. Smile and take three to five deep breaths.

7. On the last exhale, release your hands and straighten your legs. Shake your legs gently.

Variations: During the **second trimester,** you may want to modify the pose by placing a cushion under your buttocks and positioning your hands on the floor behind your hips.

During the **third trimester,** you may want to modify the pose by placing a cushion under your buttocks and sitting with your back against a wall.

Benefits: This standing pose stretches the shoulders, feet, and hips; tones the leg muscles; aligns the spine; and improves balance and posture.

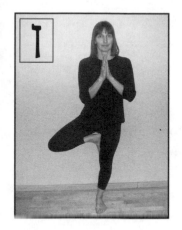

Final *Nun*—This letter is a symbol for a kingdom or a fish. A corresponding yoga pose is *vrksasana*, tree pose.

Focus/Meditation: Source of Wisdom, may my child pursue wisdom, for it is a tree of life.

How to practice the pose:

1. Stand up as straight as possible with your feet together and your arms by your sides.

2. Inhale and place your hands on your hips.

3. While still standing up straight, exhale and bend your right leg. Reach your right hand down to grasp your right ankle, balancing on your left foot.

4. Inhale and place the sole of your right foot on your left inner thigh with your toes pointing down. Press your right heel firmly into your left thigh. Press your left thigh against your right foot.

5. Exhale as you release your right ankle and bring the palms of your hands together in front of your heart. Keep your back as straight as you can. If this is an easy balance, raise your arms above your head like the branches of a tree. To help balance, focus on one spot on the wall or floor.

6. Smile and take three to five deep breaths.

7. On the last exhalation, lower your arms and right foot.

8. Repeat steps 1 through 7 on the other side.

Variations: During the **second** and **third trimesters,** you may want to modify the pose by placing one hand against a wall or on the back of a chair.

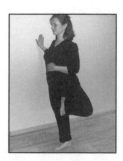

Benefits: This lying back-bending pose stretches and strengthens the thighs, lower back, shoulders, neck, and arms; improves spinal flexibility; massages the internal organs; aids digestion; and energizes the whole body.

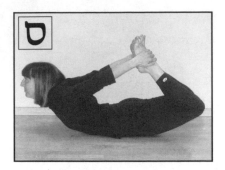

Samech—This letter is a symbol for support. A corresponding yoga pose is *dhanurasana*, bow pose.

Focus/Meditation: Merciful God, just as You remembered Sarah, Rebekah, Leah, Rachel, Bilhah, and Zilpah, protect me and help through my pregnancy.

How to practice the pose:

1. Lie flat on the floor, facing down, with your chin touching the floor and your palms by your thighs.

2. Inhale and bend both legs. Bring your feet as close to your buttocks as possible.

3. Exhale, lift your head, and reach both hands back, and grab your feet or ankles.

4. Inhale and gently raise your feet, legs, head, shoulders, and upper back as high as possible. Try to keep your knees close together.

5. Smile and take three to five deep breaths. You may find that your body rocks as you breathe. This is normal.

6. On the last exhale, release your feet and lie flat on the floor with your head turned to the right.

Cautions and Variations: *During the second and third trimesters, I suggest that you avoid this pose.* Alternatively, you may safely practice this pose while lying on your side.

Benefits: This lying pose stretches and strengthens the legs, hips, waist, biceps, and neck; and improves circulation.

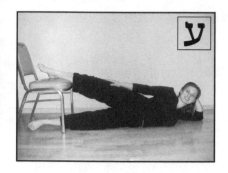

Ayin—This letter is a symbol for the eye. A corresponding yoga pose is *anantasana*, leg extension pose.

Focus/Meditation: *Shechinah*, may my child see the beauty in the world.

How to practice the pose:

1. Lie on your left side with your head propped up on your left elbow and hand.

2. Inhale and raise your right leg as as high as you can, coming to rest on a chair or block. Keep your left leg flexed straight on the floor, pushing through the heel.

3. Exhale and raise your right arm toward your right foot. Focus your gaze at your big toe or hand.

4. Smile and take three to five deep breaths.

5. On your last exhalation, lower your leg.

6. Roll onto your right side and repeat steps 1 through 5.

Cautions and Variations: As discussed earlier, *do not practice this pose during the first trimester or during the first eight weeks following delivery.*

Benefits: This back-bending pose stretches and strengthens the neck, lower back, abdomen, hips, legs, feet, and ankles; opens the throat and chest; and deepens breathing.

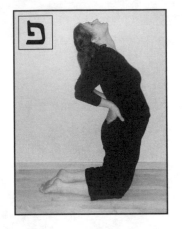

Pey—This letter is a symbol for the mouth. A corresponding yoga pose is the starting position for *ustrasana*, camel pose.

Focus/Meditation: Source of Light, may my child's mouth be full of laughter, poetry, and songs.

How to practice the pose:

1. Kneel on the floor with your thighs perpendicular to the floor.

2. Inhale and raise your right arm up. Exhale, reach back, and rest your right hand on your right hip with your fingers pointing down or to the side, away from your body.

3. Inhale and raise your left arm up. Exhale, reach back, and rest your left hand on your left hip with your fingers pointing down or to the side, away from your body.

4. Inhale and cover your top lip with your bottom lip so that you do not strain your neck. Exhale and gently lean back your head, neck, and shoulders until you are looking at the ceiling. Your hands should press your pelvis forward gently.

5. Smile (as best you can) and take three to five deep breaths.

6. Inhale and come back up to a kneeling position, perpendicular to the floor.

7. Exhale and lower your hands to your sides.

Variations: During the **second** and **third trimesters,** you can modify the pose by placing your hands or elbows on the seat of a chair behind you, rather than on your hips, for additional support.

Benefits: This standing back-bend stretches and strengthens the front torso; opens the throat and chest; expands lung capacity; and strengthens the lower back and legs.

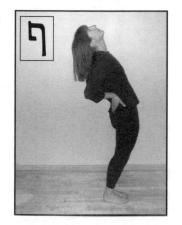

Final *Pey*—This letter is a symbol of the mouth. A corresponding yoga pose is the first step of *urdhva dhanurasana*, standing back-bend.

Focus/Meditation: My God, may the words of my mouth and the meditations of my heart be acceptable to You.

How to practice the pose:

1. Stand up as straight as possible with your arms by your sides.

2. Inhale and raise your right arm straight up. Exhale and reach back, placing your right hand on your right hip with your fingers pointing down or to the side, away from your body.

3. Inhale and raise your left arm straight up. Exhale and reach back, placing your left hand on your left hip with your fingers pointing down or to the side, away from your body.

4. Cover your top lip with your bottom lip to protect your neck, and then gently lean back your head, neck, and shoulders until you are looking at the ceiling. Your hands should press your pelvis forward gently.

5. Smile (as best as you can) and take three to five deep breaths.

6. Inhale and slowly stand up straight.

7. Exhale and release your hands.

Variations: During the **second** and **third trimesters,** you may want to modify the pose by placing hands against a wall or on the back of a chair for support.

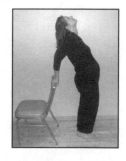

Benefits: This inverted pose strengthens the abdomen, hips, and legs; tones the waist; warms the body; massages the internal organs; and improves circulation in the feet and legs.

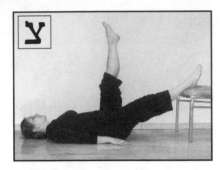

Tzadi—This letter is a symbol of righteousness or the hunt. A corresponding yoga pose is *urdhva prasarita padasana*, upright extended foot pose.

Focus/Meditation: Judge of judges, may my child be counted among the righteous.

How to practice the pose:

1. Lie flat on your back with your palms down on the floor.

2. Inhale and raise your legs together until they are perpendicular to the floor.

3. Exhale and slowly lower your right leg halfway down, coming to rest on a chair or block.

4. Smile and take three to five deep breaths.

5. On the last exhalation, lower your right leg all the way to the floor.

6. Inhale and return the right leg to a perpendicular position.

7. Repeat steps 3 through 6 with the left leg.

8. Exhale and slowly lower both legs to the floor.

Cautions and Variations: As discussed earlier, *do not practice this pose during the first trimester or during the first eight weeks following delivery.*

During the **third trimester,** you can modify the pose by placing a cushion under your buttocks, bending your knees, and lowering your legs alternately onto the seat of the chair.

Benefits: This standing pose stretches and strengthens the legs, hips, arms, and shoulders; improves balance and posture; tones the thighs; and opens the hip joints for leg mobility.

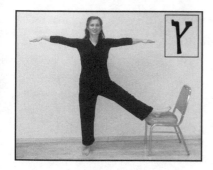

Final *Tzadi*—This letter is a symbol of righteousness or the hunt. A corresponding yoga pose is *utthita hasta padangusthasana*, extended hand and foot pose.

Focus/Meditation: Master of the universe, may my child be dedicated to performing acts of loving-kindness.

How to practice the pose:

1. Stand up as straight as possible with your arms by your sides and your left hip next to the back of a chair or windowsill that is slightly higher than your hip. Take one step to the right so that you are approximately 3 feet from the chair or windowsill.

2. Inhale and place your hands on your hips.

3. Exhale and lift your left leg sideways and carefully place your left heel on the seat of the chair or on the windowsill. If you are very flexible, grab your left big toe with your left thumb and first two fingers.

4. Inhale and raise your arms out to your sides until they are parallel to the floor. Straighten the spine, lifting up through the crown of your head. Keep both legs straight if you can. Look forward.

5. Smile and take three to five deep breaths.

6. On your last exhale, lower your arms and your leg from the chair or windowsill.

7. Repeat steps 1 through 6 on the right side.

Cautions and Variations: As discussed earlier, *do not practice this pose during the first trimester or during the first eight weeks following delivery.*

During the **third trimester,** you may want to modify the pose by leaning on a wall with one hand for support.

Benefits: This lying pose stretches the lower back, shoulders, arms, shins and ankles; massages the internal organs; and calms the mind.

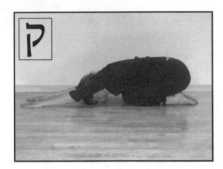

Kuf—This letter is a symbol for a monkey or to surround. A corresponding yoga pose is *pranatasana*, child's pose.

Focus/Meditation: May the Divine Presence surround and protect my child.

How to practice the pose:

1. Kneel on the floor with your buttocks touching your heels and your feet pointed backward, soles facing upward. Inhale. You may place a folded blanket under your shins for more comfortable support.

2. Exhale and lean your upper body forward until your forehead touches the floor.

3. Inhale and reach your arms forward, palms on the floor.

4. Relax and take three to five deep breaths.

5. Inhale and sit back up on your heels.

Variations: During the **second trimester,** you can modify the pose by spreading your knees as far apart as is comfortable in order to deepen the stretch in the pelvis.

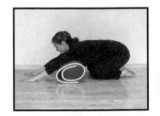

During the **third trimester,** you can modify the pose by spreading your knees and placing a stack of pillows or a rolled blanket under your chest to provide additional support and to avoid pressing directly on your belly.

Benefits: This standing pose stretches the rib cage, lower back, neck, shoulders, and waist; tones the waist; and deepens breathing.

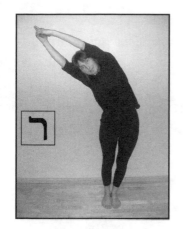

Raysh—This letter is a symbol for the head or a new beginning. A corresponding yoga pose is *nitambhasana*, reed pose.

Focus/Meditation: Source of Peace, may my child use her head to bring peace to places where there is strife.

How to practice the pose:

1. Stand up as straight as possible, feet together, with your arms by your sides.

2. Inhale and raise your arms above your head, reaching as high as you can. Try to bring your palms together while keeping your arms straight. If you are tight in your shoulders, keep your arms shoulder width apart.

3. Exhale and lean your upper body to the right as far as you can, keeping your arms straight and your biceps touching your ears. Keep your feet planted firmly on the floor; press into your heels.

4. Smile and take three to five deep breaths, stretching your side a little more with each exhalation.

5. Inhale and stand up straight.

6. Repeat steps 2 through 5 on the left side.

Variations: During the **second trimester,** you can modify the pose by lowering your arm on the side to which you lean. For example, as you lean to the right, lower your right arm and rest your right hand on your right thigh. Keep the other arm up next to your ear.

During the **third trimester,** you can modify the pose by lowering your arm and resting your hand on the back of a chair. For example, if you are leaning to the right, lower your right hand to the chair.

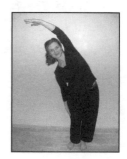

Benefits: This lying pose stretches and strengthens the neck, shoulders, arms, hips, lower back, legs, and feet; massages the internal organs; aids digestion; and energizes the whole body.

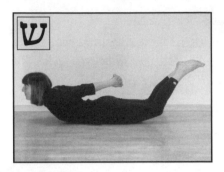

Shin—This letter is a symbol for a tooth or change. A corresponding yoga pose is *salabhasana* I, inverted boat pose.

Focus/Meditation: Eternal One, bless my child with the flexibility to bend with the changes of life.

How to practice the pose:

1. Lie flat on the floor, face down, with your feet together, your chin on the floor, and your palms on the floor by your hips.

2. Reach your hands behind your back and clasp your hands. Exhale.

3. Inhale and raise your upper body and head off the floor by pulling back with your hands. Simultaneously bend your legs, pointing your feet toward the ceiling.

4. Smile and take three to five deep breaths.

5. On the last exhalation, lower your legs and then your upper body.

6. Turn your head to the left and release your arms, placing your palms on the floor by your sides. Rest for a few breaths.

7. To come out of the pose, roll onto your right side and sit up.

Cautions and Variations: *During the second and third trimesters, you should avoid this pose.* Alternatively, you can safely modify the pose by practicing it lying on your side.

Benefits: This lying back-bending pose stretches and strengthens the abdomen, spine, and neck; provides a gentle massage to the internal organs; and aids digestion.

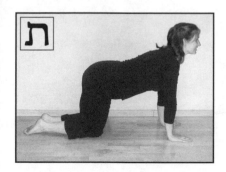

Tav—This letter is a symbol for a sign or an impression. A corresponding yoga pose is *marjarasana*, cat pose.

Focus/Meditation: Spirit of Everything, may my child's life be a sign of your love and hope for the future.

How to practice the pose:

1. Lie flat on the floor, face down.

2. Inhale and place your hands under your shoulders with your palms on the floor.

3. Exhale and push yourself up onto your hands and knees. Your arms should be straight and perpendicular to the floor.

4. Inhale deeply and look up at the ceiling, flattening your back, lengthening your stomach, and drawing your hips back toward your feet.

5. Exhale while tucking your chin to your chest, tucking your tailbone toward the floor, arching your back toward the ceiling, and pushing the air out of your lungs by contracting your stomach and diaphragm strongly. Pull your hips forward toward your arms.

6. Repeat steps 4 and 5 four more times.

Variations: During the **second** and **third trimesters,** you can modify the pose by varying the distance between your hands and knees to stretch different areas of your back.

Benefits: This twisting pose gently realigns the spine after the bending movements of the other poses. As it twists the abdomen, it massages the internal organs, helping to squeeze waste products from tissues and improve digestion.

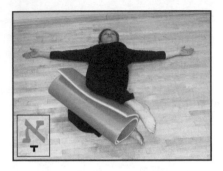

Kamatz is a Hebrew vowel with the sound "ah." A corresponding yoga pose is *jathara parivartanasana*, stomach-turning pose.

Focus/Meditation: Merciful One, may my child turn with ease within my womb.

How to practice the pose:

1. Lie flat on your back with your arms extended like a T and your feet together.

2. Inhale and raise your knees together toward your chest. Place a pillow or a rolled blanket between your knees.

3. As you exhale, slowly lower your knees to the right side, all the way to the floor if you can, but do not force it. Keep your shoulders on the floor.

4. Take a deep breath and slowly turn your head to the left. Smile and take three to five deep breaths.

5. Inhale and turn your head and knees to the center.

6. Repeat steps 3 through 5 on the other side.

Cautions and Variations: As discussed earlier, *do not practice this pose during the first trimester or during the first eight weeks following delivery.*

During the **third trimester,** I recommend placing a pillow or rolled blanket next to each knee as well as between your knees for support.

Benefits: This simple lying pose helps reduce fatigue and quiet the mind. It expands awareness of the body and breath, particularly when following the physical effort of the other poses. It helps integrate the effects of the other poses by allowing your muscles and tendons to relax completely and your breathing to return to normal.

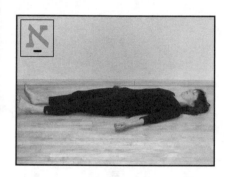

Patach is a Hebrew vowel with the sound "ah." A corresponding yoga pose is *savasana*, corpse pose.

Focus/Meditation: One who causes peace to reign in the heavens, let peace descend upon us, upon all Israel, and upon all the world.

This pose should be done at the end of every yoga session. Relax in *savasana* for 5 minutes for every half hour of practicing poses.

How to practice the pose:

1. Lie on your back with your legs about 6 inches apart, hands by your sides with your palms facing up. Close your eyes. Let your body relax into the floor.

2. Consciously slow your breathing; try to breathe so quietly that someone next to you could not hear you breathing.

3. Mentally scan your body from your feet to your face, relaxing each part of your body as you think about it. Bring your awareness to your feet and then relax your feet. Bring your awareness to your ankles. Relax your ankles. Bring your awareness to your knees and thighs. Relax your knees and thighs. Bring your awareness to your hips, lower back, and belly. Relax your hips, lower back, and belly. Bring your awareness to your upper back, shoulders, arms, elbows, and hands. Relax your upper back, shoulders, arms, elbows, and hands. Bring your awareness to your neck. Relax your neck. Bring your awareness to your scalp, face, eyes, and jaw. Relax your scalp, face, eyes, and jaw.

4. Try not to fall asleep. With your eyes closed, try to look at the inside of your forehead. Try to quiet your mind and clear it of all thoughts. Observe your breathing, the way your breath rises and falls in your belly. Let yourself melt into the floor as you relax more and more deeply. Feel your connection to the air you are breathing.

5. After at least 5 minutes, when you are ready, come out of this relaxation pose slowly. With your eyes still closed, wiggle your toes and fingers. Roll your head gently from side to side. Roll onto your right side and bend your knees so that you are in a fetal position. Take a few deep breaths. Slowly sit up to a cross-legged position. Open your eyes. Try to remember that peaceful feeling for the rest of the day. *Shalom.*

Variation: During the **second** and **third trimesters,** I recommend placing a pillow or rolled blanket under your knees. Alternatively, you may find it more comfortable to bend your knees or lie on one side in this pose.

What Is the Correct Order for Practicing Aleph-Bet Yoga during Each Trimester?

As noted earlier, the poses of Aleph-Bet Yoga should *not* be practiced in *aleph*-betical order, as they were introduced in the preceding pages. The correct order of the poses for a session is presented in the following table. Any pose that has a check mark can be done in the indicated trimester.

Name and Page Number of the Hatha Yoga Pose	Figure of the Yoga Pose	Hebrew Character	Suitable for:		
			1st TRIMESTER & POST-DELIVERY	2nd TRIMESTER	3rd TRIMESTER
1. *Tadasana*, mountain pose— see page 136 for technique.		ו	✓	✓	✓
2. *Tadasana* variation, rooster pose—see page 137 for technique.		ז	✓	✓	✓
3. *Nitambhasana*, reed pose—see page 155 for technique.		ך	✓	✓	✓
4. *Uttanasana* variation, half forward extension pose—see page 134 for technique.		ר	✓	✓	✓

Name and Page Number of the Hatha Yoga Pose	Figure of the Yoga Pose	Hebrew Character	Suitable for:		
			1st TRIMESTER & POST-DELIVERY	2nd TRIMESTER	3rd TRIMESTER
5. *Urdhva dhanurasana* variation, standing back-bend with hands on buttocks—see page 151 for technique.		ף	✓	✓	✓
6. *Tadasana* variation, mountain pose with arms extended—see page 142 for technique.		ר	✓	✓	✓
7. *Pawanmuktasana*, "wind-relieving" series for the hands and wrists—see page 140 for technique.		ד	✓	✓	✓
8. *Vrksasana*, tree pose—see page 147 for technique.		ז	✓	✓	✓
9. *Utkatasana*, lightning pose—see page 143 for technique.		ל	✓	✓	✓
10. *Virabhadrasana* variation, warrior I pose—see page 133 for technique.		ג	✓	✓	✓

Name and Page Number of the Hatha Yoga Pose	Figure of the Yoga Pose	Hebrew Character	Suitable for:		
			1ST TRIMESTER & POST-DELIVERY	2ND TRIMESTER	3RD TRIMESTER
11. *Utthita trikonasana*, extended triangle pose—see page 131 for technique.		א	✓	✓	✓
12. *Ardha chandrasana*, half-moon pose—see page 138 for technique.		ח	✓	✓	✓
13. *Prasarita padottanasana* variation, extended foot pose—see page 135 for technique.		ה	✓	✓	✓
14. *Utthita hasta padangusthasana*, extended hand and foot pose—see page 153 for technique.		צ	X*	✓	✓
15. *Dandasana* variation, stick pose with arms extended and with *pawanmuktasana*, "wind relieving" series for the feet and ankles—see page 132 for technique.		ב	✓	✓	✓
16. *Janu sirsasana* variation, knee-head pose—see page 141 for technique.	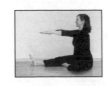	כ	✓	✓	✓

* Do not include in series during this trimester.

Name and Page Number of the Hatha Yoga Pose	Figure of the Yoga Pose	Hebrew Character	Suitable for: 1ST TRIMESTER & POST-DELIVERY	2ND TRIMESTER	3RD TRIMESTER
17. *Paschimottanasana*, seated forward bend—see page 145 for technique.	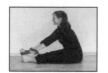	ס	X*	✓	✓
18. *Badha konasana*, butterfly or cobbler pose—see page 146 for technique.		נ		✓	✓	✓
19. *Ardha navasana*, half-boat pose—see page 139 for technique.		ט		✓	✓	✓
20. *Urdhva prasarita padasana* variation, upright extended foot pose—see page 152 for technique.	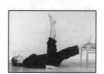	צ	X*	✓	✓
21. *Anantasana*, leg extension pose—see page 149 for technique.	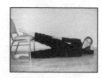	ע	X*	✓	✓
22. *Ustrasana* variation, camel pose with hands on buttocks—see page 150 for technique.		פ		✓	✓	✓

* Do not include in series during this trimester.

Name and Page Number of the Hatha Yoga Pose	Figure of the Yoga Pose	Hebrew Character	Suitable for:		
			1ST TRIMESTER & POST-DELIVERY	2ND TRIMESTER	3RD TRIMESTER
23. *Ustrasana* variation, camel pose with hands on floor—see page 144 for technique.	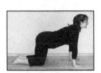		✓	✓	✓
24. *Marjarasana*, cat pose— see page 157 for technique.	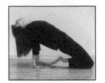		✓	✓	✓
25. *Salabhasana* I, inverted boat pose— see page 156 for technique.	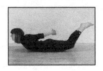		✓	X*	X*
26. *Dhanurasana*, bow pose— see page 148 for technique.	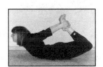		✓	X*	X*
27. *Pranatasana*, child's pose— see page 154 for technique.	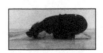		✓	✓	✓
28. *Jathara parivartanasana*, stomach-turning pose— see page 158 for technique.	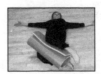		X*	✓	✓
29. *Savasana*, corpse pose— see page 159 for technique.	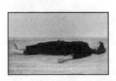		✓	✓	✓

* Do not include in series during this trimester.

Guidelines for a Shorter Session

Practicing all the poses in the series should take approximately 30 to 40 minutes. If you are pressed for time, use the following guidelines for an alternative session that takes about 20 minutes.

For a shorter session **in the first trimester or during the two-month period of recovery following delivery, I suggest the following alternatives to the full series:**

- Choose one or more of the three standing poses that are based on the mountain pose (*vav*, *zayin*, or final *kaf*), instead of doing all three in one session.
- Do all the poses for *raysh*, *dalet*, final *pey*, *yud*, final *nun*, *lamed*, and *gimmel*.
- Choose either *aleph* or *chet* pose.
- Do *hay* but not final *tzadi* pose.
- Choose either *mem* or *kaf* for a sitting forward-bending pose but do not do final *mem* pose.
- Do *nun* pose, but do not do *tet* pose.
- Choose either *pey* or *mem* pose.
- Do *tav* pose.
- Choose either *shin* or *samech* pose.
- Finish with *kuf*, followed by *patach* pose.

For a shorter session during the second or third trimesters:

- Choose one or more of the three standing poses that are based on the mountain pose (*vav*, *zayin*, or final *kaf*) instead of doing all three in one session.
- Do all of the poses for *raysh*, *dalet*, final *pey*, *yud*, final *nun*, *lamed*, and *gimmel*.
- Choose either *aleph* or *chet* pose.
- Choose either *hay* or final *tzadi* pose.
- Choose one or more of the three sitting forward-bending poses (final *mem*, *bet*, or *kaf*).

- Do *nun* and *tet* pose.
- Choose either *pey* or *mem* pose.
- Do *tav* pose.
- Skip the poses for *shin* and *samech*.
- Finish with *kuf* pose, followed by *kamatz* and *patach* poses.

Notes

Chapter 1 • The First Trimester

1. Blu Greenberg, *How to Run a Traditional Jewish Household* (New York: Simon & Schuster, 1983), 236.

2. G. Samsioe and G. M. Veliner, "Nausea and Vomiting in Pregnancy—A Contribution to Its Epidemiology," *Gynecology Obstetrical Investigations* 16 (1983): 221–229.

3. R. M. Weigel and M. M. Weigel, "Nausea and Vomiting of Early Pregnancy and Pregnancy Outcome: A Meta-Analytical Review," *British Journal of Obstetrics and Gynecology* 96 (1989):1312–1318.

4. V. Sahakian, D. Rouse, and S. Sipes, et al., "Vitamin B6 Is Effective Therapy for Nausea and Vomiting of Pregnancy: A Randomized, Double-Blind Placebo-Controlled Study," *Obstetrics and Gynecology* 78 (1991): 33–36.

5. P. Mazzotta and L. A. Magee, "A Risk-Benefit Assessment of Pharmacological and Nonpharmacological Treatments for Nausea and Vomiting of Pregnancy," *Drugs* 59 (2000): 781–800.

6. "Rabbi" is a talmudic figure who is referred to without a name, only as "Rabbi."

7. See E. E. Urbach, *The Sages: Their Concepts and Beliefs*, trans. by Israel Abrahams (Cambridge, Mass.: Harvard University Press, 1979), 242ff.

8. David Feldman, *Marital Relations, Birth Control and Abortion in Jewish Law* (New York: Schocken Books, 1974), 273.

9. "*Seder Yetzirat Ha-vlad* (Treatise on the Formation of the Embryo)," translated in Raphael Patai, *Gates of the Old City: A Book of Jewish Legends* (New York: Avon Books, 1980), 378–381.

10. A. J. Wilcox, C. R. Weinberg, J. F. O'Connor, et al., "Incidence of Early Pregnancy Loss," *New England Journal of Medicine* 319 (1988):189–194.

11. Michelle Klein, *A Time to Be Born: Customs and Folklore of Jewish Birth* (Philadelphia: Jewish Publication Society, 2000), 105–106.

12. Julius Preuss, *Biblical and Talmudic Medicine*, trans. and ed. by Fred Rosner (Northvale, N.J. Jason Aronson, 1993), 385.

13. Klein, *A Time to Be Born*, 111.

14. Nina Beth Cardin, *Out of the Depths I Call to You: A Book of Prayers for the Married Jewish Woman* (Northvale, N.J.: Jason Aronson, 1992), 72–77.

Chapter 2 • The Second Trimester

1. S. Harlap and P. H. Shiono, "Alcohol, Smoking, and Incidence of Spontaneous Abortions in the First and Second Trimester," *Lancet* 2 (1973, 1980a.): 173–176.

2. American College of Obstetricians and Gynecologists (ACOG), American College of Medical Genetics, *Preconception and Prenatal Carrier Screening for Cystic Fibrosis* (Washington, D.C.: ACOG, 2001).

3. ACOG, *Screening for Tay-Sachs Disease* (Washington, D.C.: ACOG, 1995).

4. ACOG, *Screening for Canavan Disease* (Washington, D.C.: ACOG, 1998).

5. J. David Bleich, "Abortion in Halakhic Literature," in *Jewish Bioethics*, edited by Fred Rosner and David Bleich (New York: Sanhedrin Press, 1979), 135.

6. Quoted in Fred Rosner's "Tay-Sachs Disease: To Screen or Not to Screen" in *Jewish Bioethics*, edited by Fred Rosner and J. David Bleich (New York: Sanhedrin Press, 1979), 179.

7. The following discussion is taken from Elliot Dorff, *Matters of Life and Death: A Jewish Approach to Modern Medical Ethics*, (Philadelphia: Jewish Publication Society, 1998), 128–133.

8. Ibid., 131.

9. Ibid., 132.

10. Walter Jacob, "When Is Abortion Permitted?" *Contemporary American Reform Responsa* (New York: CCAR Press, 1987), 23–27.

11. Jacob Emden, *Sh'eilat Ya'avetz*, No. 43.

12. W. Gunther Plaut and Dr. Mark Washovsky, "Abortion to Save Sibling from Suffering," *Teshuvot for the 1990s* (New York: CCAR Press, 1997), 173.

13. J. A. Martin, B. E. Hamilton, F. Menacker, M. M. Park, *Births: Final Data for 2000* 50:2. (Hyattsville, Md.: National Vital Statistics Reports, 2002).

14. This ceremony is rarely performed in the liberal Jewish community, though there are some who still perform it in some way. The ceremony is done only for the mother's firstborn child who was delivered vaginally, not through Cesarean section. The reason is because the Torah refers specifically to the first child born of the opening of the womb (Exodus 13:2).

15. Dorff, *Matters of Life and Death*, 129–130.

16. Ladino, a mixture of Spanish and Hebrew, is a dialect spoken by some Sephardic Jews.

17. Rabbi Rifat Sonsino, born and raised in Turkey, remembers that "the cutting of the swaddling clothes" was done for all pregnancies, not just the first one.

18. Klein, *A Time to Be Born*, 86.

Chapter 3 • The Third Trimester

1. Cardin, *Out of the Depths I Call to You*, 78–84.
2. Translation by Nina Beth Cardin in *Tears of Sorrow, Seeds of Hope* (Woodstock, Vt.: Jewish Lights Publishing, 1999),123.
3. See pages 15–16 for a more detailed description of the red thread from Rachel's Tomb.
4. Cardin, *Out of the Depths I Call to You*, 100–103.
5. It should be further noted that the story of Yael has a connection with birthing. The story is read every year in synagogue as the Haftarah, the accompaniment, to the reading of the Song at the Sea from the Book of Exodus. This story of Israel's miraculous crossing of the Red Sea will be discussed in the next chapter as a powerful birthing image.
6. M. B. Stephens, L. A. Fenton, and S. A. Fields, "Obstetric Analgesia," *Primary Care: Clinics in Office Practice* 27 (2000): 203–220.
7. The blessing was written by the Creative Ritual Team at Mayyim Chayyim, the Boston mikvah. It was written specifically for using the mikvah for noncommanded occasions. Commanded occasions, such as after menstruation and conversion, are specified as obligatory by Jewish law.
8. R. L. Copper, et al., "A Multicenter Study of Preterm Birth Weight and Gestational Age-Specific Mortality," *American Journal of Obstetrics and Gynecology* 168 (1993):78.

Chapter 4 • Labor and Delivery

1. Fanny Neruda, "Prayer on the Approach of Accouchement," trans. from the German by M. Mayer, reprinted in *Sarah's Daughters Sing: A Sampler of Poems by Jewish Women*, Henny Wenkart, ed. (Hoboken, N.J.: KTAV Publishing, 1990), 140–141.

2. M. Mongelli, M. Wilcox, J. Gardosi, "Estimating the Date of Confinement: Ultrasonographic Biometry versus Certain Menstrual Dates," *American Journal of Obstetrics and Gynecology* 174 (1996): 278–281.

3. R. L. Copper, et al., "A Multicenter Study," 78.

4. Preuss, *Biblical and Talmudic Medicine*, 393.

5. Naomi Rusk shared this insight with us.

6. Preuss, *Biblical and Talmudic Medicine*, 394.

7. See Raphael Patai, *On Jewish Folklore* (Detroit: Wayne State University Press, 1983), 337–446, for a full description of these customs.

8. In Kurdistan, the shofar would be blown right next to the laboring woman, "so that the names of certain angels should penetrate the woman's ears," cited in Patai, *On Jewish Folklore*, 380.

9. Patai, *On Jewish Folklore*, 380–381.

10. For an etrog to be fit for use during Sukkot, it must have its end (pitom). When the pitom is bitten off, the etrog becomes unfit for the mitzvah of shaking the lulav and the etrog.

11. Chava Weissler, "Mitzvot Built into the Body; Tkhines for Niddah, Pregnancy, and Childbirth," in *People of the Body: Jews and Judaism from an Embodied Perspective*, edited by Howard Eilberg-Schwartz (Albany: State University of New York Press, 1992), 108–109.

12. Tikva Frymer-Kensky, *Motherprayer: The Pregnant Women's Spiritual Companion* (New York: Riverhead Books, 1995), 182.

13. Cardin, *Out of the Depths I Call to You*, 100.

14. *Reconstructionist Rabbinical Association Rabbi's Manual* (Wyncote, Penn.: 1997), 5. The capitalization of the names of God are from the manual.

15. J. Naveh and S. Shaked, *Magic Spells and Formulae* (Jerusalem: Magnes Press, 1993), 147.

16. Patai, *On Jewish Folklore*, 392.

Chapter 5 • The Days after Birth

1. *Reconstructionist Rabbinical Association Rabbi's Manual*, 11.
2. For more information about Shalom Zachar, see Blu Greenberg's *How to Run a Traditional Jewish Household*, 240.
3. *The Alphabet of Ben Sira*, as quoted in *Which Lilith?*, Enid Dame, Lilly Rivlin, and Henny Wenkart, eds. (Northvale, N.J.: Jason Aronson, 1998), 7.
4. This essay is adapted from an article that first appeared in *Lilith*, 27, no. 3 (2002): 27–30.
5. I. Yalom, D. Lunde, R. Moos, et al., "Postpartum Blues Syndrome," *Archives of General Psychiatry* 18 (1968): 16–27.
6. *Shulkhan Aruch, Orach Chayim* 219: 9.
7. Rochelle Millen, "Birkat Ha-Gomel: A Study in Cultural Context and Halakhic Practice," *Judaism* 43 (1994): 270–278.

Chapter 6 • From This Narrow Place
I Call to You: Pregnancy Loss

1. A. J. Wilcox, C. R. Weinberg, J. F. O'Connor, et al., "Incidence of Early Pregnancy Loss," *New England Journal of Medicine* 319 (1988): 189.
2. Adapted from Amy Eilberg, "A Grieving Ritual Following Miscarriage or Stillbirth," in *Lifecycles, Vol. 1: Jewish Women on Life Passages & Personal Milestones*, edited by Debra Orenstein (Woodstock, Vt.: Jewish Lights Publishing, 1994), 48–51.

Glossary

B'rit Bat: The covenant ceremony for a girl. It can occur on a day of one's choosing.

B'rit Milah: The circumcision ceremony that occurs on the eighth day after birth.

Halakhah: Jewish law.

Kavvana: Intention.

Midrash; plural, midrashim: A rabbinic story, parable, or interpretation of biblical text, coming from the root *d-r-sh*, which means "to examine." Midrashim help fill in gaps in the text, supply missing details or dialogue, and enliven the text with anecdotes. Early midrashim can be found in the Talmud, from the second century, but the first actual compendia were edited in the fifth and sixth centuries C.E. Modern midrashim are still being written today.

Mikvah; **plural,** *mikvaot:* A pool of water used for ritual immersions containing both natural rainwater and tap water, built and filled to exact legal specifications. *Mikvaot* are used traditionally to immerse new dishes, brides (and in some cases grooms), converts to Judaism, and women after their menstrual periods. They have also been used during the ninth month of pregnancy, after a miscarriage, and after a birth.

Mishnah: A collection of legal decisions edited in the third century C.E. Considered the first work of Jewish law, the Mishnah also forms the basis for the Talmud (see below).

Mitzvah; **plural,** *mitzvot:* Commandments; good deeds.

Pidyon haben: A ceremony performed thirty days after birth of the firstborn son of the mother. The ceremony involves "buying back" the child from God via a *kohain* (a person of Jewish priestly lineage), usually for five silver coins.

Rabbis: The term "the Rabbis" refers to the Rabbis whose stories, conversations, and legal decisions are recorded in the Talmud.

Responsum: Jewish legal opinion.

Shviti: A traditional Jewish art form used for meditation.

Talmud: The compilation of rabbinic law, comprising the Mishnah (see above) and the Gemara (rabbinic discussions of the Mishnah, edited in the sixth century C.E.)

Further Resources

Pregnancy

Cardin, Nina Beth. *Out of the Depths I Call to You: A Book of Prayers for the Married Jewish Woman*. Northvale, N.J.: Jason Aronson, 1995.

Frymer-Kensky, Tikva. *Motherprayer: The Pregnant Woman's Spiritual Companion*. New York: Riverhead Books, 1995.

Klein, Michelle. *A Time to Be Born: Customs and Folklore of Jewish Birth*. Philadelphia: Jewish Publication Society, 1998.

Klirs, Tracy Guren, ed. *The Merit of Our Mothers: A Bilingual Anthology of Jewish Women's Prayers*. Cincinnati, Ohio: Hebrew Union College Press, 1992.

Orenstein, Debra, ed. *Lifecycles Volume 1: Jewish Women on Life Passages and Personal Milestones*. Woodstock, Vt.: Jewish Lights Publishing, 1994.

Pregnancy Loss

Cardin, Rabbi Nina Beth. *Tears of Sorrow, Seeds of Hope: A Jewish Companion for Infertility and Pregnancy Loss*. Woodstock, Vt.: Jewish Lights Publishing, 1999.

Kohn, Ingrid, Perry-Lynn Moffitt, Isabelle A. Wilkins, and Michael Berman. *A Silent Sorrow: Pregnancy Loss—Guidance and Support for You and Your Family*. New York: Routledge, 2000.

Jewish Bio-Medical Ethics

Dorff, Elliot. *Matters of Life and Death: A Jewish Approach to Modern Medical Ethics*. Philadelphia: Jewish Publication Society, 1998.

Feldman, Emanuel, and Joel Wolowelsky, eds. *Jewish Law and the New Reproductive Technologies*. Hoboken, N.J.: KTAV, 1998.

Rosner, Fred, and J. David Bleich, eds. *Jewish Bioethics*. New York: Sanhedrin Press, 1979.

Jewish Covenant Rituals

Breger, Jennifer, and Lisa Schlaff. *The Orthodox Jewish Women and Ritual: Options and Opportunities*. New York: Jewish Orthodox Feminist Alliance, 2000.

Cohen, Debra Nussbaum. *Celebrating Your New Jewish Daughter: Creating Jewish Ways to Welcome Baby Girls into the Covenant*. Woodstock, Vt.: Jewish Lights Publishing, 2001.

Diamant, Anita. *The New Jewish Baby Book: Names, Ceremonies & Customs—A Guide for Today's Families*. Woodstock, Vt.: Jewish Lights Publishing, 1994.

Rituals for Jewish Childbirth. http://ritualwell.org.

Yoga

Books

Balaskas, Janet. *Preparing for Birth with Yoga*. Rockport, Mass.: Element Books, 1994.

Iyengar, Geeta. *Yoga: A Gem for Women*. Spokane, Wash.: Timeless Books, 1990.

Rapp, Steven A. *Aleph-Bet Yoga: Embodying the Hebrew Letters for Physical and Spiritual Well-Being*. Woodstock, Vt.: Jewish Lights Publishing, 2002.

Video

Yoga Journal's Prenatal Yoga with Shiva Rea. Broomfield, Colo.: Gaiam, 2000.

Jewish Parenting

Abramowitz, Yosef, and Susan Silverman. *Jewish Family & Life: Traditions, Holidays, and Values for Today's Parents and Children*. New York: Golden Books, 1997.

Abrams, Rabbi Judith, and Dr. Steven Abrams. *Jewish Parenting: Rabbinic Insights*. Northvale, N.J.: Jason Aronson, 1994.

Diamant, Anita, with Karen Kushner. *How to Be a Jewish Parent: A Practical Handbook for Family Life*. New York: Schocken Books, 2000.

Fuchs-Kreimer, Rabbi Nancy. *Parenting as a Spiritual Journey Deepening Ordinary & Extraordinary Events into Sacred Occasions*. Woodstock, Vt.: Jewish Lights Publishing, 1998.

Gordis, Daniel. *Becoming a Jewish Parent: How to Explore Spirituality and Tradition with Your Children*. New York: Three Rivers Press, 1999.

Mogul, Wendy. *The Blessing of a Skinned Knee: Using Jewish Teachings to Raise Self-Reliant Children*. New York: Penguin Compass, 2001.

The New Jewish Baby Album: Creating and Celebrating the Beginning of a Spiritual Life—A Jewish Lights Companion. Edited by Jewish Lights. Woodstock, Vt.: Jewish Lights Publishing, 2003.

Rosman, Steve. *Jewish Parenting Wisdom*. Northvale, N.J.: Jason Aronson, 1997.

Grateful acknowledgement is given for permission to use material from the following sources:

Amy Bardack, for permission to print *"Birkat Hagomel,"* © 2004 by Amy Bardack.

Franci Levine Grater, for permission to print "Twins in NICU," © 2004 by Franci Levine Grater.

Rabbi Susan Silverman, for permission to print "Prayer Before an Amniocentesis" and "Prayer Before an Ultrasound," © 2004 by Rabbi Susan Silverman.

Aurora Mendelsohn, for permission to reprint "Breastfeeding," © 2002 by Aurora Mendelsohn, which first appeared as part of an expanded version in the fall 2002 issue of *Lilith: The Independent Jewish Woman's Magazine*, and permission to print "Prayer for a Newborn Child," © 2004 by Aurora Mendelsohn.

Richard Hirsh, for permission to reprint "Prayer for Bringing a Child Home for the First Time" and "Prayer for a Safe Delivery," © 1997 by the Reconstructionist Rabbinical Association. Reprinted from the RRA Rabbi's Manual.

Sandy Eisenberg Sasso, for permission to print "Prayer upon Learning of a Pregnancy," © 2004 by Sandy Eisenberg Sasso.

Jewish Lights Publishing, for permission to reprint "A Prayer for the Husband to Say When His Wife Is Pregnant," from *Tears of Sorrow, Seeds of Hope: A Jewish Spiritual Companion for Infertility and Pregnancy Loss* © 1999 by Nina Beth Cardin (Woodstock, Vt.: Jewish Lights Publishing). $19.95 + $3.75s/h. Order by mail or call 800-962-4544 or on-line at www.jewishlights.com. Permission is granted by Jewish Lights Publishing, P.O. Box 237, Woodstock, VT 05091.

Amy Friedman, for permission to print "Visiting the *Mikvah* in the Ninth Month," © 2004 by Amy Friedman.

Rabbi Michelle Robinson, for permission to print "It Better Be a Sister," © 2004 by Rabbi Michelle Robinson.

Sandy Slavet, for permission to print "Prayer for Carrying a Fetus with a Problem," © 2004 by Sandy Slavet.

Joanna Selznick Dulkin, for permission to print "Preparing to Be a Jewish Parent," © 2004 by Joanna Selznick Dulkin.

Martha Hausman, for permission to print "Praying for a Good *Neshama* (Soul)," © 2004 by Martha Hausman.

Rabbi Shohama Wiener, for permission to print "A Birthing Support Ritual," © 2004 by Rabbi Shohama Wiener.

Jewish Lights Publishing, for permission to reprint "A Grieving Ritual Following Miscarriage or Stillbirth" by Amy Eilberg in *Lifecycles, Vol 1: Jewish Women on Life Passages and Personal Milestones*, edited by Deborah Orenstein, © 1994 by Deborah Orenstein (Woodstock, Vt.: Jewish Lights Publishing). $19.95 + $3.75s/h. Order by mail or call 800-962-4544 or on-line at www.jewishlights.com. Permission is granted by Jewish Lights Publishing, P.O. Box 237, Woodstock, VT 05091.

Jason Aronson, for permission to reprint from *Out of the Depths I Call to You: A Book of Prayers for the Married Jewish Woman* by Nina Beth Cardin, © 1992 by Nina Beth Cardin (Northvale NJ: Jason Aronson).

Maqom: A School for Adult Talmud Study, for permission to reprint the *shviti* image.

Index

Bar/Bat Mitzvah

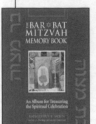

The Bar/Bat Mitzvah Memory Book
An Album for Treasuring the Spiritual Celebration
By Rabbi Jeffrey K. Salkin and Nina Salkin
A unique album for preserving the spiritual memories of the day, and for recording plans for the Jewish future ahead. Contents include space for creating or recording family history; teachings received from rabbi, cantor, and others; mitzvot and *tzedakot* chosen and carried out, etc.
8 x 10, 48 pp, Deluxe Hardcover, 2-color text, ribbon marker, ISBN 1-58023-111-X **$19.95**

Bar/Bat Mitzvah Basics: A Practical Family Guide to Coming of Age Together
Edited by Helen Leneman. Foreword by Rabbi Jeffrey K. Salkin.
6 x 9, 240 pp, Quality PB, ISBN 1-58023-151-9 **$18.95**

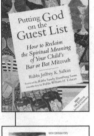

For Kids—Putting God on Your Guest List: How to Claim the Spiritual Meaning of Your Bar or Bat Mitzvah *By Rabbi Jeffrey K. Salkin*
6 x 9, 144 pp, Quality PB, ISBN 1-58023-015-6 **$14.95** *For ages 11–12*

Putting God on the Guest List: How to Reclaim the Spiritual Meaning of Your Child's Bar or Bat Mitzvah *By Rabbi Jeffrey K. Salkin*
6 x 9, 224 pp, Quality PB, ISBN 1-879045-59-1 **$16.95**

Tough Questions Jews Ask: A Young Adult's Guide to Building a Jewish Life
By Rabbi Edward Feinstein 6 x 9, 160 pp, Quality PB, ISBN 1-58023-139-X **$14.95** *For ages 13 & up*
Also Available: **Tough Questions Jews Ask Teacher's Guide**
8½ x 11, 72 pp, PB, ISBN 1-58023-187-X **$8.95**

Bible Study/Midrash

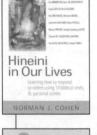

Hineini in Our Lives: Learning How to Respond to Others through 14 Biblical Texts, and Personal Stories *By Norman J. Cohen*
6 x 9, 240 pp, Hardcover, ISBN 1-58023-131-4 **$23.95**

Ancient Secrets: Using the Stories of the Bible to Improve Our Everyday Lives
By Rabbi Levi Meier, Ph.D. 5½ x 8½, 288 pp, Quality PB, ISBN 1-58023-064-4 **$16.95**

Moses—The Prince, the Prophet His Life, Legend & Message for Our Lives
By Rabbi Levi Meier, Ph.D.
6 x 9, 224 pp, Quality PB, ISBN 1-58023-069-5 **$16.95**; Hardcover, ISBN 1-58023-013-X **$23.95**

Self, Struggle & Change: Family Conflict Stories in Genesis and Their Healing Insights for Our Lives *By Norman J. Cohen* 6 x 9, 224 pp, Quality PB, ISBN 1-879045-66-4 **$16.95**

Voices from Genesis: Guiding Us through the Stages of Life *By Norman J. Cohen*
6 x 9, 192 pp, Quality PB, ISBN 1-58023-118-7 **$16.95**

Congregation Resources

Becoming a Congregation of Learners: Learning as a Key to Revitalizing Congregational Life *By Isa Aron, Ph.D. Foreword by Rabbi Lawrence A. Hoffman.*
6 x 9, 304 pp, Quality PB, ISBN 1-58023-089-X **$19.95**

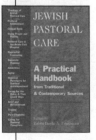

Finding a Spiritual Home: How a New Generation of Jews Can Transform the American Synagogue *By Rabbi Sidney Schwarz*
6 x 9, 352 pp, Quality PB, ISBN 1-58023-185-3 **$19.95**

Jewish Pastoral Care: A Practical Handbook from Traditional & Contemporary Sources
Edited by Rabbi Dayle A. Friedman 6 x 9, 464 pp, Hardcover, ISBN 1-58023-078-4 **$35.00**

The Self-Renewing Congregation: Organizational Strategies for Revitalizing Congregational Life *By Isa Aron, Ph.D. Foreword by Dr. Ron Wolfson.*
6 x 9, 304 pp, Quality PB, ISBN 1-58023-166-7 **$19.95**

Or phone, fax, mail or e-mail to: **JEWISH LIGHTS Publishing**
Sunset Farm Offices, Route 4 • P.O. Box 237 • Woodstock, Vermont 05091
Tel: (802) 457-4000 • Fax: (802) 457-4004 • www.jewishlights.com
Credit card orders: (800) 962-4544 (8:30AM–5:30PM ET Monday–Friday)
Generous discounts on quantity orders. SATISFACTION GUARANTEED. Prices subject to change.

Children's Books

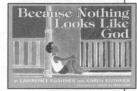

Because Nothing Looks Like God
By Lawrence and Karen Kushner

What is God like? The first collaborative work by husband-and-wife team Lawrence and Karen Kushner introduces children to the possibilities of spiritual life. Real-life examples of happiness and sadness invite us to explore, together with our children, the questions we all have about God, no matter what our age.

11 x 8½, 32 pp, Full-color illus., Hardcover, ISBN 1-58023-092-X **$16.95** *For ages 4 & up*

Also Available: **Because Nothing Looks Like God Teacher's Guide**
8½ x 11, 22 pp, PB, ISBN 1-58023-140-3 **$6.95** *For ages 5–8*

Board Book Companions to *Because Nothing Looks Like God*
5 x 5, 24 pp, Full-color illus., SkyLight Paths Board Books, **$7.95** each *For ages 0–4*

What Does God Look Like? ISBN 1-893361-23-3

How Does God Make Things Happen? ISBN 1-893361-24-1

Where Is God? ISBN 1-893361-17-9

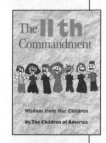

The 11th Commandment: Wisdom from Our Children
by The Children of America

"If there were an Eleventh Commandment, what would it be?" Children of many religious denominations across America answer this question—in their own drawings and words.

8 x 10, 48 pp, Full-color illus., Hardcover, ISBN 1-879045-46-X **$16.95** *For all ages*

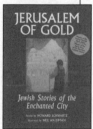

Jerusalem of Gold: Jewish Stories of the Enchanted City
Retold by Howard Schwartz. Full-color illus. by Neil Waldman.

A beautiful and engaging collection of historical and legendary stories for children. Each celebrates the magical city that has served as a beacon for the Jewish imagination for three thousand years. Draws on Talmud, midrash, Jewish folklore, and mystical and Hasidic sources.

8 x 10, 64 pp, Full-color illus., Hardcover, ISBN 1-58023-149-7 **$18.95** *For ages 7 & up*

The Book of Miracles: A Young Person's Guide to Jewish Spiritual Awareness
By Lawrence Kushner. All-new illustrations by the author.

6 x 9, 96 pp, 2-color illus., Hardcover, ISBN 1-879045-78-8 **$16.95** *For ages 9–13*

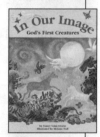

In Our Image: God's First Creatures
By Nancy Sohn Swartz

9 x 12, 32 pp, Full-color illus., Hardcover, ISBN 1-879045-99-0 **$16.95** *For ages 4 & up*

From SKYLIGHT PATHS PUBLISHING

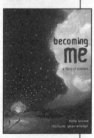

Becoming Me: A Story of Creation
By Martin Boroson. Full-color illus. by Christopher Gilvan-Cartwright.

Told in the personal "voice" of the Creator, a story about creation and relationship that is about each one of us. In simple words and with radiant illustrations, the Creator tells an intimate story about love, about friendship and playing, about our world—and about ourselves.

8 x 10, 32 pp, Full-color illus., Hardcover, ISBN 1-893361-11-X **$16.95** *For ages 4 & up*

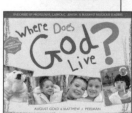

Ten Amazing People: And How They Changed the World
By Maura D. Shaw. Foreword by Dr. Robert Coles. Full-color illus. by Stephen Marchesi.

Black Elk • Dorothy Day • Malcolm X • Mahatma Gandhi • Martin Luther King, Jr. • Mother Teresa • Janusz Korczak • Desmond Tutu • Thich Nhat Hanh • Albert Schweitzer • This vivid, inspirational, and authoritative book will open new possibilities for children by telling the stories of how ten of the past century's greatest leaders changed the world in important ways.

8½ x 11, 48 pp, Full-color illus., Hardcover, ISBN 1-893361-47-0 **$17.95** *For ages 7 & up*

Where Does God Live? *By August Gold and Matthew J. Perlman*

Using simple, everyday examples that children can relate to, this colorful book helps young readers develop a personal understanding of God.

10 x 8½ , 32 pp, Full-color photo illus., Quality PB, ISBN 1-893361-39-X **$8.95** *For ages 3–6*

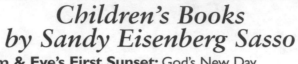

Children's Books
by Sandy Eisenberg Sasso

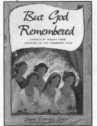

Adam & Eve's First Sunset: God's New Day

Engaging new story explores fear and hope, faith and gratitude in ways that will delight kids and adults—inspiring us to bless each of God's days and nights.

9 x 12, 32 pp, Full-color illus., Hardcover, ISBN 1-58023-177-2 **$17.95** *For ages 4 & up*

But God Remembered

Stories of Women from Creation to the Promised Land

Four different stories of women—Lillith, Serach, Bityah, and the Daughters of Z—teach us important values through their faith and actions.

9 x 12, 32 pp, Full-color illus., Hardcover, ISBN 1-879045-43-5 **$16.95** *For ages 8 & up*

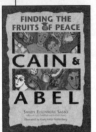

Cain & Abel: Finding the Fruits of Peace

Full-color illus. by Joani Keller Rothenberg

Shows children that we have the power to deal with anger in positive ways. Provides questions for kids and adults to explore together.

9 x 12, 32 pp, Full-color illus., Hardcover, ISBN 1-58023-123-3 **$16.95** *For ages 5 & up*

God in Between

Full-color illus. by Sally Sweetland

If you wanted to find God, where would you look? This magical, mythical tale teaches that God can be found where we are: within all of us and the relationships between us.

9 x 12, 32 pp, Full-color illus., Hardcover, ISBN 1-879045-86-9 **$16.95** *For ages 4 & up*

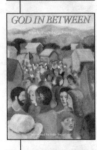

God's Paintbrush

Wonderfully interactive, invites children of all faiths and backgrounds to encounter God through moments in their own lives. Provides questions adult and child can explore together.

11 x 8½, 32 pp, Full-color illus., Hardcover, ISBN 1-879045-22-2 **$16.95** *For ages 4 & up*

Also Available: **God's Paintbrush Teacher's Guide**

8½ x 11, 32 pp, PB, ISBN 1-879045-57-5 **$8.95**

God's Paintbrush Celebration Kit

A Spiritual Activity Kit for Teachers and Students of All Faiths, All Backgrounds
Additional activity sheets available:
8-Student Activity Sheet Pack (40 sheets/5 sessions), ISBN 1-58023-058-X **$19.95**
Single-Student Activity Sheet Pack (5 sessions), ISBN 1-58023-059-8 **$3.95**

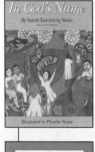

In God's Name

Full-color illus. by Phoebe Stone

Like an ancient myth in its poetic text and vibrant illustrations, this award-winning modern fable about the search for God's name celebrates the diversity and, at the same time, the unity of all people.

9 x 12, 32 pp, Full-color illus., Hardcover, ISBN 1-879045-26-5 **$16.95** *For ages 4 & up*

Also Available as a Board Book: **What Is God's Name?**

5 x 5, 24 pp, Board, Full-color illus., ISBN 1-893361-10-1 **$7.95** *For ages 0–4 (A SkyLight Paths book)*

Also Available: **In God's Name video and study guide**

Computer animation, original music, and children's voices. 18 min. **$29.99**

Also Available in Spanish: **El nombre de Dios**

9 x 12, 32 pp, Full-color illus., Hardcover, ISBN 1-893361-63-2 **$16.95** *(A SkyLight Paths book)*

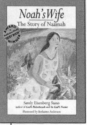

Noah's Wife: The Story of Naamah

When God tells Noah to bring the animals of the world onto the ark, God also calls on Naamah, Noah's wife, to save each plant on Earth. Based on an ancient text.

9 x 12, 32 pp, Full-color illus., Hardcover, ISBN 1-58023-134-9 **$16.95** *For ages 4 & up*

Also Available as a Board Book: **Naamah, Noah's Wife**

5 x 5, 24 pp, Full-color illus., Board, ISBN 1-893361-56-X **$7.95** *For ages 0–4 (A SkyLight Paths book)*

For Heaven's Sake: Finding God in Unexpected Places

9 x 12, 32 pp, Full-color illus., Hardcover, ISBN 1-58023-054-7 **$16.95** *For ages 4 & up*

God Said Amen: Finding the Answers to Our Prayers

9 x 12, 32 pp, Full-color illus., Hardcover, ISBN 1-58023-080-6 **$16.95** *For ages 4 & up*

Abraham Joshua Heschel

The Earth Is the Lord's: The Inner World of the Jew in Eastern Europe
5½ x 8, 128 pp, Quality PB, ISBN 1-879045-42-7 **$14.95**

Israel: An Echo of Eternity *New Introduction by Susannah Heschel*
5½ x 8, 272 pp, Quality PB, ISBN 1-879045-70-2 **$19.95**

A Passion for Truth: Despair and Hope in Hasidism
5½ x 8, 352 pp, Quality PB, ISBN 1-879045-41-9 **$18.95**

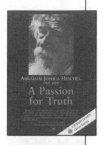

Holidays/Holy Days

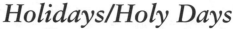

7th Heaven: Celebrating Shabbat with Rebbe Nachman of Breslov
By Moshe Mykoff with the Breslov Research Institute
Based on the teachings of Rebbe Nachman of Breslov. Explores the art of consciously observing Shabbat and understanding in-depth many of the day's traditional spiritual practices.
5⅛ x 8¼, 224 pp, Deluxe PB w/flaps, ISBN 1-58023-175-6 **$18.95**

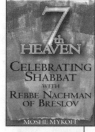

The Women's Passover Companion
Women's Reflections on the Festival of Freedom
Edited by Rabbi Sharon Cohen Anisfeld, Tara Mohr, and Catherine Spector
A groundbreaking collection that captures the voices of Jewish women who engage in a provocative conversation about women's relationships to Passover as well as the roots and meanings of women's seders.
6 x 9, 352 pp, Hardcover, ISBN 1-58023-128-4 **$24.95**

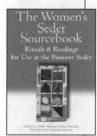

The Women's Seder Sourcebook
Rituals & Readings for Use at the Passover Seder
Edited by Rabbi Sharon Cohen Anisfeld, Tara Mohr, and Catherine Spector
This practical guide gathers the voices of more than one hundred women in readings, personal and creative reflections, commentaries, blessings, and ritual suggestions that can be incorporated into your Passover celebration as supplements to or substitutes for traditional passages of the haggadah.
6 x 9, 384 pp, Hardcover, ISBN 1-58023-136-5 **$24.95**

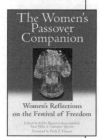

Hanukkah, 2nd Edition: The Family Guide to Spiritual Celebration
By Dr. Ron Wolfson. Edited by Joel Lurie Grishaver.
7 x 9, 240 pp, illus., Quality PB, ISBN 1-58023-122-5 **$18.95**

The Jewish Gardening Cookbook: Growing Plants & Cooking for
Holidays & Festivals *By Michael Brown*
6 x 9, 224 pp, 30+ illus., Quality PB, ISBN 1-58023-116-0 **$16.95**;
Hardcover, ISBN 1-58023-004-0 **$21.95**

Passover, 2nd Edition: The Family Guide to Spiritual Celebration
By Dr. Ron Wolfson with Joel Lurie Grishaver
7 x 9, 352 pp, Quality PB, ISBN 1-58023-174-8 **$19.95**

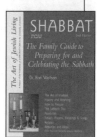

Shabbat, 2nd Edition: The Family Guide to Preparing for and Celebrating the Sabbath
By Dr. Ron Wolfson 7 x 9, 320 pp, illus., Quality PB, ISBN 1-58023-164-0 **$19.95**

Sharing Blessings: Children's Stories for Exploring the Spirit of the Jewish Holidays
By Rahel Musleah and Michael Klayman
8½ x 11, 64 pp, Full-color illus., Hardcover, ISBN 1-879045-71-0 **$18.95** *For ages 6 & up*

The Jewish Family Fun Book: Holiday Projects, Everyday Activities, and Travel Ideas with Jewish Themes
By Danielle Dardashti and Roni Sarig. Illus. by Avi Katz.
With almost 100 easy-to-do activities to re-invigorate age-old Jewish customs and make them fun for the whole family, this complete sourcebook details activities for fun at home and away from home, including meaningful everyday and holiday crafts, recipes, travel guides, enriching entertainment and much, much more. Illustrated.
6 x 9, 288 pp, 70+ b/w illus. & diagrams, Quality PB, ISBN 1-58023-171-3 **$18.95**

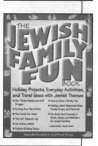

Life Cycle
Parenting

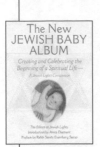

The New Jewish Baby Album: Creating and Celebrating the Beginning of a Spiritual Life—A Jewish Lights Companion
By the Editors at Jewish Lights. Foreword by Anita Diamant. Preface by Sandy Eisenberg Sasso.
A spiritual keepsake that will be treasured for generations. More than just a memory book, *shows you how—and why it's important*—to create a Jewish home and a Jewish life. Includes sections to describe naming ceremony, space to write encouragements, and pages for writing original blessings, prayers, and meaningful quotes throughout.
8 x 10, 64 pp, Deluxe Padded Hardcover, Full-color illus., ISBN 1-58023-138-1 **$19.95**

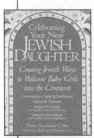

The Jewish Pregnancy Book: A Resource for the Soul, Body & Mind during Pregnancy, Birth & the First Three Months
By Dr. Sandy Falk, M.D., and Rabbi Daniel Judson, with Steven A. Rapp
Includes medical information on fetal development, pre-natal testing and more, from a liberal Jewish perspective; prenatal *aleph-bet* yoga; and ancient and modern prayers and rituals for each stage of pregnancy.
7 x 10, 144 pp, Quality PB, Layflat binding, b/w illus., ISBN 1-58023-178-0 **$16.95**

Celebrating Your New Jewish Daughter: Creating Jewish Ways to Welcome Baby Girls into the Covenant—New and Traditional Ceremonies
By Debra Nussbaum Cohen 6 x 9, 272 pp, Quality PB, ISBN 1-58023-090-3 **$18.95**

The New Jewish Baby Book: Names, Ceremonies & Customs—A Guide for Today's Families *By Anita Diamant* 6 x 9, 336 pp, Quality PB, ISBN 1-879045-28-1 **$18.95**

Parenting As a Spiritual Journey: Deepening Ordinary and Extraordinary Events into Sacred Occasions *By Rabbi Nancy Fuchs-Kreimer*
6 x 9, 224 pp, Quality PB, ISBN 1-58023-016-4 **$16.95**

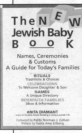

Embracing the Covenant: Converts to Judaism Talk About Why & How
Edited and with introductions by Rabbi Allan Berkowitz and Patti Moskovitz
6 x 9, 192 pp, Quality PB, ISBN 1-879045-50-8 **$16.95**

The Guide to Jewish Interfaith Family Life: An InterfaithFamily.com Handbook
Edited by Ronnie Friedland and Edmund Case 6 x 9, 384 pp, Quality PB, ISBN 1-58023-153-5 **$18.95**

Making a Successful Jewish Interfaith Marriage: The Jewish Outreach Institute Guide to Opportunities, Challenges and Resources
By Rabbi Kerry Olitzky with Joan Peterson Littman 6 x 9, 176 pp, Quality PB, ISBN 1-58023-170-5 **$16.95**

The Perfect Stranger's Guide to Wedding Ceremonies
A Guide to Etiquette in Other People's Religious Ceremonies *Edited by Stuart M. Matlins*
6 x 9, 208 pp, Quality PB, ISBN 1-893361-19-5 **$16.95** *(A SkyLight Paths book)*

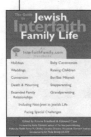

How to Be a Perfect Stranger, 3rd Edition
The Essential Religious Etiquette Handbook
Edited by Stuart M. Matlins and Arthur J. Magida
The indispensable guidebook to help the well-meaning guest when visiting other people's religious ceremonies.
A straightforward guide to the rituals and celebrations of the major religions and denominations in the United States and Canada from the perspective of an interested guest of any other faith, based on information obtained from authorities of each religion. Belongs in every living room, library, and office.
6 x 9, 432 pp, Quality PB, ISBN 1-893361-67-5 **$19.95** *(A SkyLight Paths book)*

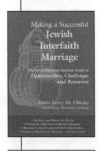

Divorce Is a Mitzvah: A Practical Guide to Finding Wholeness and Holiness When Your Marriage Dies *By Rabbi Perry Netter. Afterword by Rabbi Laura Geller.*
6 x 9, 224 pp, Quality PB, ISBN 1-58023-172-1 **$16.95**

A Heart of Wisdom: Making the Jewish Journey from Midlife through the Elder Years
Edited by Susan Berrin. Foreword by Harold Kushner. 6 x 9, 384 pp, Quality PB, ISBN 1-58023-051-2 **$18.95**

So That Your Values Live On: Ethical Wills and How to Prepare Them
Edited by Jack Riemer and Nathaniel Stampfer 6 x 9, 272 pp, Quality PB, ISBN 1-879045-34-6 **$18.95**

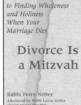

Meditation

The Handbook of Jewish Meditation Practices
A Guide for Enriching the Sabbath and Other Days of Your Life
By Rabbi David A. Cooper
Easy-to-learn meditation techniques for use on the Sabbath and every day, to help us return to the roots of traditional Jewish spirituality where Shabbat is a state of mind and soul. 6 x 9, 208 pp, Quality PB, ISBN 1-58023-102-0 **$16.95**

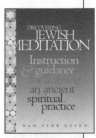

Discovering Jewish Meditation: Instruction & Guidance for Learning an Ancient Spiritual Practice *By Nan Fink Gefen, Ph.D.* 6 x 9, 208 pp, Quality PB, ISBN 1-58023-067-9 **$16.95**

A Heart of Stillness: A Complete Guide to Learning the Art of Meditation
By Rabbi David A. Cooper
5½ x 8½, 272 pp, Quality PB, ISBN 1-893361-03-9 **$16.95** *(A SkyLight Paths book)*

Meditation from the Heart of Judaism: Today's Teachers Share Their Practices, Techniques, and Faith *Edited by Avram Davis*
6 x 9, 256 pp, Quality PB, ISBN 1-58023-049-0 **$16.95**

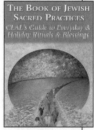

Silence, Simplicity & Solitude: A Complete Guide to Spiritual Retreat at Home
By Rabbi David A. Cooper
5½ x 8½, 336 pp, Quality PB, ISBN 1-893361-04-7 **$16.95** *(A SkyLight Paths book)*

Three Gates to Meditation Practice: A Personal Journey into Sufism, Buddhism, and Judaism *By Rabbi David A. Cooper*
5½ x 8½, 240 pp, Quality PB, ISBN 1-893361-22-5 **$16.95** *(A SkyLight Paths book)*

The Way of Flame: A Guide to the Forgotten Mystical Tradition of Jewish Meditation
By Avram Davis 4½ x 6, 176 pp, Quality PB, ISBN 1-58023-060-1 **$15.95**

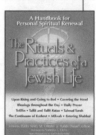

Ritual/Sacred Practice

The Jewish Dream Book
The Key to Opening the Inner Meaning of Your Dreams
By Vanessa L. Ochs with Elizabeth Ochs; Full-color Illus. by Kristina Swarner
Vibrant illustrations, instructions for how modern people can perform ancient Jewish dream practices, and dream interpretations drawn from the Jewish wisdom tradition help make this guide the ideal bedside companion for anyone who wants to further their understanding of their dreams—and themselves.
8 x 8, 120 pp, Full-color illus., Deluxe PB w/flaps, ISBN 1-58023-132-2 **$16.95**

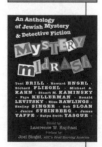

The Rituals & Practices of a Jewish Life: A Handbook for Personal Spiritual Renewal *Edited by Rabbi Kerry M. Olitzky and Rabbi Daniel Judson*
6 x 9, 272 pp, illus., Quality PB, ISBN 1-58023-169-1 **$18.95**

The Book of Jewish Sacred Practices: CLAL's Guide to Everyday & Holiday Rituals & Blessings *Edited by Rabbi Irwin Kula and Vanessa L. Ochs, Ph.D.*
6 x 9, 368 pp, Quality PB, ISBN 1-58023-152-7 **$18.95**

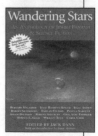

Science Fiction/ Mystery & Detective Fiction

Mystery Midrash: An Anthology of Jewish Mystery & Detective Fiction
Edited by Lawrence W. Raphael. Preface by Joel Siegel.
6 x 9, 304 pp, Quality PB, ISBN 1-58023-055-5 **$16.95**

Criminal Kabbalah: An Intriguing Anthology of Jewish Mystery & Detective Fiction
Edited by Lawrence W. Raphael. Foreword by Laurie R. King.
6 x 9, 256 pp, Quality PB, ISBN 1-58023-109-8 **$16.95**

More Wandering Stars: An Anthology of Outstanding Stories of Jewish Fantasy and Science Fiction *Edited by Jack Dann. Introduction by Isaac Asimov.*
6 x 9, 192 pp, Quality PB, ISBN 1-58023-063-6 **$16.95**

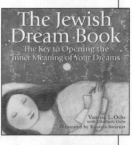

Wandering Stars: An Anthology of Jewish Fantasy & Science Fiction
Edited by Jack Dann. Introduction by Isaac Asimov.
6 x 9, 272 pp, Quality PB, ISBN 1-58023-005-9 **$16.95**

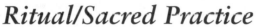

Spirituality

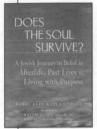

The Alphabet of Paradise: An A–Z of Spirituality for Everyday Life
By Rabbi Howard Cooper
In twenty-six engaging chapters, Cooper spiritually illuminates the subjects of our daily lives—A to Z—examining these sources by using an ancient Jewish mystical method of interpretation that reveals both the literal and more allusive meanings of each.   5 x 7¾, 224 pp, Quality PB, ISBN 1-893361-80-2 **$16.95** *(A SkyLight Paths book)*

Does the Soul Survive?: A Jewish Journey to Belief in Afterlife, Past Lives & Living with Purpose   *By Rabbi Elie Kaplan Spitz. Foreword by Brian L Weiss, M.D.*
Spitz relates his own experiences and those shared with him by people he has worked with as a rabbi, and shows us that belief in afterlife and past lives, so often approached with reluctance, is in fact true to Jewish tradition.
6 x 9, 288 pp, Quality PB, ISBN 1-58023-165-9 **$16.95**; Hardcover, ISBN 1-58023-094-6 **$21.95**

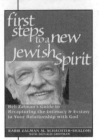

First Steps to a New Jewish Spirit: Reb Zalman's Guide to Recapturing the Intimacy & Ecstasy in Your Relationship with God
By Rabbi Zalman M. Schachter-Shalomi with Donald Gropman
An extraordinary spiritual handbook that restores psychic and physical vigor by introducing us to new models and alternative ways of practicing Judaism. Offers meditation and contemplation exercises for enriching the most important aspects of everyday life.   6 x 9, 144 pp, Quality PB, ISBN 1-58023-182-9 **$16.95**

God in Our Relationships: Spirituality between People from the Teachings of Martin Buber   *By Rabbi Dennis S. Ross*
On the eightieth anniversary of Buber's classic work, we can discover new answers to critical issues in our lives. Inspiring examples from Ross's own life—as congregational rabbi, father, hospital chaplain, social worker, and husband—illustrate Buber's difficult-to-understand ideas about how we encounter God and each other. 5½ x 8½, 160 pp, Quality PB, ISBN 1-58023-147-0 **$16.95**

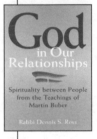

The Jewish Lights Spirituality Handbook: A Guide to Understanding, Exploring & Living a Spiritual Life   *Edited by Stuart M. Matlins*
What exactly is "Jewish" about spirituality? How do I make it a part of my life? Fifty of today's foremost spiritual leaders share their ideas and experience with us.
6 x 9, 456 pp, Quality PB, ISBN 1-58023-093-8 **$19.95**; Hardcover, ISBN 1-58023-100-4 **$24.95**

Bringing the Psalms to Life: How to Understand and Use the Book of Psalms
By Dr. Daniel F. Polish
6 x 9, 208 pp, Quality PB, ISBN 1-58023-157-8 **$16.95**; Hardcover, ISBN 1-58023-077-6 **$21.95**

God & the Big Bang: Discovering Harmony between Science & Spirituality
By Dr. Daniel C. Matt 6 x 9, 216 pp, Quality PB, ISBN 1-879045-89-3 **$16.95**

Godwrestling—Round 2: Ancient Wisdom, Future Paths
By Rabbi Arthur Waskow 6 x 9, 352 pp, Quality PB, ISBN 1-879045-72-9 **$18.95**

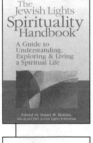

One God Clapping: The Spiritual Path of a Zen Rabbi   *By Rabbi Alan Lew with Sherril Jaffe*
5½ x 8½, 336 pp, Quality PB, ISBN 1-58023-115-2 **$16.95**

The Path of Blessing: Experiencing the Energy and Abundance of the Divine
By Rabbi Marcia Prager 5½ x 8½, 240 pp., Quality PB, ISBN 1-58023-148-9 **$16.95**

Six Jewish Spiritual Paths: A Rationalist Looks at Spirituality   *By Rabbi Rifat Sonsino*
6 x 9, 208 pp, Quality PB, ISBN 1-58023-167-5 **$16.95**; Hardcover, ISBN 1-58023-095-4 **$21.95**

Soul Judaism: Dancing with God into a New Era
By Rabbi Wayne Dosick 5½ x 8½, 304 pp, Quality PB, ISBN 1-58023-053-9 **$16.95**

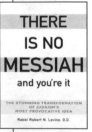

Stepping Stones to Jewish Spiritual Living: Walking the Path Morning, Noon, and Night   *By Rabbi James L. Mirel and Karen Bonnell Werth*
6 x 9, 240 pp, Quality PB, ISBN 1-58023-074-1 **$16.95**; Hardcover, ISBN 1-58023-003-2 **$21.95**

There Is No Messiah... and You're It: The Stunning Transformation of Judaism's Most Provocative Idea   *By Rabbi Robert N. Levine, D.D.*
6 x 9, 192 pp, Hardcover, ISBN 1-58023-173-X **$21.95**

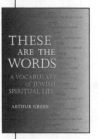

These Are the Words: A Vocabulary of Jewish Spiritual Life   *By Dr. Arthur Green*
6 x 9, 304 pp, Quality PB, ISBN 1-58023-107-1 **$18.95**

Spirituality/Lawrence Kushner

The Book of Letters: A Mystical Hebrew Alphabet
Popular Hardcover Edition, 6 x 9, 80 pp, 2-color text, ISBN 1-879045-00-1 **$24.95**
Deluxe Gift Edition with slipcase, 9 x 12, 80 pp, 4-color text, Hardcover, ISBN 1-879045-01-X **$79.95**
Collector's Limited Edition, 9 x 12, 80 pp, gold foil embossed pages, w/limited edition silkscreened
print, ISBN 1-879045-04-4 **$349.00**

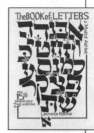

The Book of Miracles: A Young Person's Guide to Jewish Spiritual Awareness
All-new illustrations by the author
6 x 9, 96 pp, 2-color illus., Hardcover, ISBN 1-879045-78-8 **$16.95** *For ages 9–13*

The Book of Words: Talking Spiritual Life, Living Spiritual Talk
6 x 9, 160 pp, Quality PB, ISBN 1-58023-020-2 **$16.95**

Eyes Remade for Wonder: A Lawrence Kushner Reader
Introduction by Thomas Moore
6 x 9, 240 pp, Quality PB, ISBN 1-58023-042-3 **$18.95;** Hardcover, ISBN 1-58023-014-8 **$23.95**

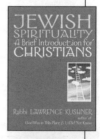

God Was in This Place & I, i Did Not Know
Finding Self, Spirituality and Ultimate Meaning
6 x 9, 192 pp, Quality PB, ISBN 1-879045-33-8 **$16.95**

Honey from the Rock: An Introduction to Jewish Mysticism
6 x 9, 176 pp, Quality PB, ISBN 1-58023-073-3 **$16.95**

Invisible Lines of Connection: Sacred Stories of the Ordinary
5½ x 8½, 160 pp, Quality PB, ISBN 1-879045-98-2 **$15.95**

Jewish Spirituality—A Brief Introduction for Christians
5¼ x 8¼, 112 pp, Quality PB Original, ISBN 1-58023-150-0 **$12.95**

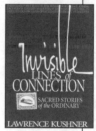

The River of Light: Jewish Mystical Awareness
6 x 9, 192 pp, Quality PB, ISBN 1-58023-096-2 **$16.95**

The Way Into Jewish Mystical Tradition
6 x 9, 224 pp, Hardcover, ISBN 1-58023-029-6 **$21.95**

Spirituality/Prayer

Pray Tell: A Hadassah Guide to Jewish Prayer
By Rabbi Jules Harlow, with contributions from Tamara Cohen, Rochelle Furstenberg, Rabbi Daniel Gordis, Leora Tanenbaum, and many others
A guide to traditional Jewish prayer enriched with insight and wisdom from a broad variety of viewpoints—from Orthodox, Conservative, Reform, and Reconstructionist Judaism to New Age and feminist. Offers fresh and modern slants on what it means to pray as a Jew, and how women and men might actually pray. 8½ x 11, 400 pp, Quality PB, ISBN 1-58023-163-2 **$29.95**

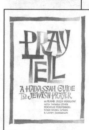

My People's Prayer Book Series
Traditional Prayers, Modern Commentaries
Edited by Rabbi Lawrence A. Hoffman
Provides diverse and exciting commentary to the traditional liturgy, helping modern men and women find new wisdom in Jewish prayer, and bring liturgy into their lives. Each book includes Hebrew text, modern translation, and commentaries from all perspectives of the Jewish world.

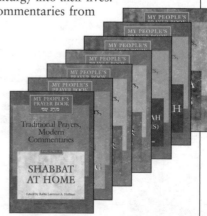

Vol. 1—The *Sh'ma* and Its Blessings
7 x 10, 168 pp, Hardcover, ISBN 1-879045-79-6 **$23.95**
Vol. 2—The *Amidah*
7 x 10, 240 pp, Hardcover, ISBN 1-879045-80-X **$24.95**
Vol. 3—*P'sukei D'zimrah* (Morning Psalms)
7 x 10, 240 pp, Hardcover, ISBN 1-879045-81-8 **$24.95**
Vol. 4—*Seder K'riat Hatorah* (The Torah Service)
7 x 10, 264 pp, Hardcover, ISBN 1-879045-82-6 **$23.95**
Vol. 5—*Birkhot Hashachar* (Morning Blessings)
7 x 10, 240 pp, Hardcover, ISBN 1-879045-83-4 **$24.95**
Vol. 6—*Tachanun* and Concluding Prayers
7 x 10, 240 pp, Hardcover, ISBN 1-879045-84-2 **$24.95**
Vol. 7—Shabbat at Home
7 x 10, 240 pp, Hardcover, ISBN 1-879045-85-0 **$24.95**

Spirituality/The Way Into... Series

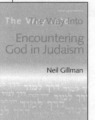

The Way Into... Series offers an accessible and highly usable "guided tour" of the Jewish faith, people, history and beliefs—in total, an introduction to Judaism that will enable you to understand and interact with the sacred texts of the Jewish tradition. Each volume is written by a leading contemporary scholar and teacher, and explores one key aspect of Judaism. *The Way Into...* enables all readers to achieve a real sense of Jewish cultural literacy through guided study.

The Way Into Encountering God in Judaism *By Neil Gillman*
6 x 9, 240 pp, Hardcover, ISBN 1-58023-025-3 **$21.95**

Also Available: **The Jewish Approach to God: A Brief Introduction for Christians**
By Neil Gillman 5½ x 8½, 192 pp, Quality PB, ISBN 1-58023-190-X **$16.95**

The Way Into Jewish Mystical Tradition *By Lawrence Kushner*
6 x 9, 224 pp, Hardcover, ISBN 1-58023-029-6 **$21.95**

The Way Into Jewish Prayer *By Lawrence A. Hoffman*
6 x 9, 224 pp, Hardcover, ISBN 1-58023-027-X **$21.95**

The Way Into Torah *By Norman J. Cohen*
6 x 9, 176 pp, Hardcover, ISBN 1-58023-028-8 **$21.95**

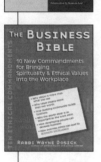

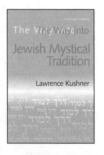

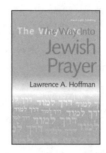

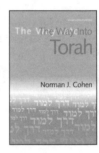

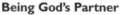

Spirituality in the Workplace

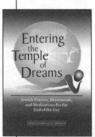

Being God's Partner
How to Find the Hidden Link Between Spirituality and Your Work
By Rabbi Jeffrey K. Salkin. Introduction by Norman Lear.
6 x 9, 192 pp, Quality PB, ISBN 1-879045-65-6 **$17.95**

The Business Bible: 10 New Commandments for Bringing Spirituality & Ethical Values into the Workplace *By Rabbi Wayne Dosick*
5½ x 8½, 208 pp, Quality PB, ISBN 1-58023-101-2 **$14.95**

Spirituality and Wellness

Aleph-Bet Yoga
Embodying the Hebrew Letters for Physical and Spiritual Well-Being
By Steven A. Rapp. Foreword by Tamar Frankiel, Ph.D., and Judy Greenfeld. Preface by Hart Lazer
7 x 10, 128 pp, b/w photos, Quality PB, Layflat binding, ISBN 1-58023-162-4 **$16.95**

Entering the Temple of Dreams
Jewish Prayers, Movements, and Meditations for the End of the Day
By Tamar Frankiel, Ph.D., and Judy Greenfeld
7 x 10, 192 pp, illus., Quality PB, ISBN 1-58023-079-2 **$16.95**

Minding the Temple of the Soul
Balancing Body, Mind, and Spirit through Traditional Jewish Prayer, Movement, and Meditation
By Tamar Frankiel, Ph.D., and Judy Greenfeld
7 x 10, 184 pp, illus., Quality PB, ISBN 1-879045-64-8 **$16.95**
Audiotape of the Blessings and Meditations: 60 min. **$9.95**
Videotape of the Movements and Meditations: 46 min. **$20.00**

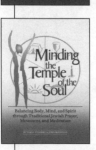

Spirituality/Women's Interest

Lifecycles, Vol. 1: Jewish Women on Life Passages & Personal Milestones
Edited and with introductions by Rabbi Debra Orenstein
6 x 9, 480 pp, Quality PB, ISBN 1-58023-018-0 **$19.95**

Lifecycles, Vol. 2: Jewish Women on Biblical Themes in Contemporary Life
Edited and with introductions by Rabbi Debra Orenstein and Rabbi Jane Rachel Litman
6 x 9, 464 pp, Quality PB, ISBN 1-58023-019-9 **$19.95**

Moonbeams: A Hadassah Rosh Hodesh Guide *Edited by Carol Diament, Ph.D.*
8½ x 11, 240 pp, Quality PB, ISBN 1-58023-099-7 **$20.00**

ReVisions: Seeing Torah through a Feminist Lens *By Rabbi Elyse Goldstein*
5½ x 8½, 224 pp, Quality PB, ISBN 1-58023-117-9 **$16.95**

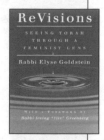

White Fire: A Portrait of Women Spiritual Leaders in America
By Rabbi Malka Drucker. Photographs by Gay Block.
7 x 10, 320 pp, 30+ b/w photos, Hardcover, ISBN 1-893361-64-0 **$24.95** *(A SkyLight Paths book)*

Women of the Wall: Claiming Sacred Ground at Judaism's Holy Site
Edited by Phyllis Chesler and Rivka Haut
6 x 9, 496 pp, b/w photos, Hardcover, ISBN 1-58023-161-6 **$34.95**

The Women's Torah Commentary: New Insights from Women Rabbis on the 54
Weekly Torah Portions *Edited by Rabbi Elyse Goldstein*
6 x 9, 496 pp, Hardcover, ISBN 1-58023-076-8 **$34.95**

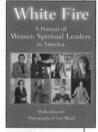

The Year Mom Got Religion: One Woman's Midlife Journey into Judaism
By Lee Meyerhoff Hendler
6 x 9, 208 pp, Quality PB, ISBN 1-58023-070-9 **$15.95**; Hardcover, ISBN 1-58023-000-8 **$19.95**

See Holidays for *The Women's Passover Companion: Women's Reflections on
the Festival of Freedom* and *The Women's Seder Sourcebook: Rituals &
Readings for Use at the Passover Seder.*

Theology/Philosophy

Aspects of Rabbinic Theology
By Solomon Schechter. New Introduction by Dr. Neil Gillman.
6 x 9, 448 pp, Quality PB, ISBN 1-879045-24-9 **$19.95**

Broken Tablets: Restoring the Ten Commandments and Ourselves
Edited by Rachel S. Mikva. Introduction by Lawrence Kushner. Afterword by Arnold Jacob Wolf.
6 x 9, 192 pp, Quality PB, ISBN 1-58023-158-6 **$16.95**; Hardcover, ISBN 1-58023-066-0 **$21.95**

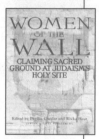

Creating an Ethical Jewish Life
A Practical Introduction to Classic Teachings on How to Be a Jew
By Dr. Byron L. Sherwin and Seymour J. Cohen
6 x 9, 336 pp, Quality PB, ISBN 1-58023-114-4 **$19.95**

The Death of Death: Resurrection and Immortality in Jewish Thought
By Dr. Neil Gillman 6 x 9, 336 pp, Quality PB, ISBN 1-58023-081-4 **$18.95**

Evolving Halakhah: A Progressive Approach to Traditional Jewish Law
By Rabbi Dr. Moshe Zemer
6 x 9, 480 pp, Quality PB, ISBN 1-58023-127-6 **$29.95**; Hardcover, ISBN 1-58023-002-4 **$40.00**

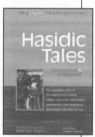

Hasidic Tales: Annotated & Explained
By Rabbi Rami Shapiro. Foreword by Andrew Harvey, SkyLight Illuminations series editor.
5½ x 8½, 192 pp, Quality PB, ISBN 1-893361-86-1 **$16.95** *(A SkyLight Paths Book)*

A Heart of Many Rooms: Celebrating the Many Voices within Judaism
By Dr. David Hartman
6 x 9, 352 pp, Quality PB, ISBN 1-58023-156-X **$19.95**; Hardcover, ISBN 1-58023-048-2 **$24.95**

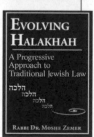

Judaism and Modern Man: An Interpretation of Jewish Religion
By Will Herberg. New Introduction by Dr. Neil Gillman.
5½ x 8½, 336 pp, Quality PB, ISBN 1-879045-87-7 **$18.95**

Keeping Faith with the Psalms: Deepen Your Relationship with God Using the
Book of Psalms *By Daniel F. Polish*
6 x 9, 272 pp, Hardcover, ISBN 1-58023-179-9 **$24.95**

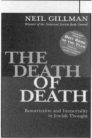

About Jewish Lights

People of all faiths and backgrounds yearn for books that attract, engage, educate, and spiritually inspire.

Our principal goal is to stimulate thought and help all people learn about who the Jewish People are, where they come from, and what the future can be made to hold. While people of our diverse Jewish heritage are the primary audience, our books speak to people in the Christian world as well and will broaden their understanding of Judaism and the roots of their own faith.

We bring to you authors who are at the forefront of spiritual thought and experience. While each has something different to say, they all say it in a voice that you can hear.

Our books are designed to welcome you and then to engage, stimulate, and inspire. We judge our success not only by whether or not our books are beautiful and commercially successful, but by whether or not they make a difference in your life.

For your information and convenience, at the back of this book we have provided a list of other Jewish Lights books you might find interesting and useful. They cover all the categories of your life:

Bar/Bat Mitzvah	Life Cycle
Bible Study / Midrash	Meditation
Children's Books	Parenting
Congregation Resources	Prayer
Current Events / History	Ritual / Sacred Practice
Ecology	Spirituality
Fiction: Mystery, Science Fiction	Theology / Philosophy
Grief / Healing	Travel
Holidays / Holy Days	Twelve Steps
Inspiration	Women's Interest
Kabbalah / Mysticism / Enneagram	

Stuart M. Matlins, Publisher

Or phone, fax, mail or e-mail to: **JEWISH LIGHTS Publishing**
Sunset Farm Offices, Route 4 • P.O. Box 237 • Woodstock, Vermont 05091
Tel: (802) 457-4000 • Fax: (802) 457-4004 • www.jewishlights.com
Credit card orders: **(800) 962-4544** (8:30AM–5:30PM ET Monday–Friday)
Generous discounts on quantity orders. SATISFACTION GUARANTEED. Prices subject to change.

For more information about each book, visit our website at www.jewishlights.com